PUBLIC HEALTH: PRACTICES, METHODS AND POLICIES

CHILD ENVIRONMENTAL HEALTH DISPARITIES

LOOKING AT THE PRESENT AND FACING THE FUTURE

PUBLIC HEALTH: PRACTICES, METHODS AND POLICIES

JOAV MERRICK - SERIES EDITOR

MEDICAL DIRECTOR, HEALTH SERVICES, DIVISION FOR INTELLECTUAL AND DEVELOPMENTAL DISABILITIES, MINISTRY OF SOCIAL AFFAIRS AND SOCIAL SERVICES, JERUSALEM, ISRAEL

Child Environmental Health Disparities: Looking at the Present and Facing the Future
I. Leslie Rubin and Joav Merrick (Editors)
2020. ISBN: 978-1-53617-823-4 (Hardcover)

Positive Youth Development: Digital Game-Based Learning
Ty Lee, Daniel T.L. Shek, Sarah Sw Lee, and Joav Merrick (Editors)
2020. ISBN: 978-1-53617-795-4 (Hardcover)

Service Leadership Education in an Era of Service Economy
Daniel TL Shek, Xiaoqin Zhu, and Joav Merrick (Editors)
2020. ISBN: 978-1-53617-514-1 (Hardcover)
2020. ISBN: 978-1-53617-515-8 (e-book)

Parenting and Family Life in a Chinese Society
Daniel TL Shek, Moon YM Law, Joav Merrick (Editors)
2020. ISBN: 978-1-53616-705-4 (Softcover)
2020. ISBN: 978-1-53616-706-1 (e-book)

Public Health: Topics, Themes and Trends
Satesh Bidaisee, Sadik Uddin Emmanuel Keku, Joav Merrick (Editors)
2020. ISBN: 978-1-53616-655-2 (Softcover)
2020. ISBN: 978-1-53616-656-9

Public Health: Environment and Child Health in a Changing World
I. Leslie Rubin and Joav Merrick (Editors)
2019. ISBN: 978-1-53615-394-1 (Hardcover)
2019. ISBN: 978-1-53615395-8 (e-book)

Service Leadership: Tools to Assess Knowledge, Attitude and Behavior
Daniel TL Shek, Xiaoqin Zhu, Li Lin and Joav Merrick (Editors)
2019. ISBN: 978-1-53614-852-7 (Hardcover)
2019. ISBN: 978-1-53614-853-4 (e-book)

Public Health Yearbook 2017
Joav Merrick (Editor)
2018. ISBN: 978-1-53613-792-7 (Hardcover)
2018. ISBN: 978-1-53613-793-4 (e-book)

Resilience and Health: A Potent Dynamic
I Leslie Rubin and Joav Merrick (Editors)
2018. ISBN: 978-1-53613-412-4 (Hardcover)
2018. ISBN: 978-1-53613-413-1 (e-book)

Medical History: Some Perspectives Second Edition
Donald E. Greydanus and Joav Merrick, (Editors)
2018. ISBN: 978-1-53613-319-6 (Hardcover)
2018. ISBN: 978-1-53613-320-2 (e-book)

University Students: Promotion of Holistic Development in Hong Kong
Daniel TL Shek, Lu Yu and Joav Merrick (Editors)
2017. ISBN: 978-1-53612-535-1 (Hardcover)
2017. ISBN: 978-1-53612-537-5 (e-book)

Alzheimer's Disease: Awareness among Young Adults
Ronald Chow, Drew Hollenberg, Michael Borean and Joav Merrick (Editors)
2017. ISBN: 978-1-53612-456-9 (Softcover)
2017. ISBN: 978-1-53612-457-6 (e-book)

Service Leadership Education for University Students
Daniel TL Shek, Po Chung, Li Lin and Joav Merrick (Editors)
2017. ISBN: 978-1-53611-949-7 (Hardcover)
2017. ISBN: 978-1-53611-969-5 (e-book)

Leadership: Promoting Leadership and Intrapersonal Development in University Students
Daniel TL Shek, Cecilia MS Ma and Joav Merrick (Editors)
2017. ISBN: 978-1-53611-950-3 (Hardcover)
2017. ISBN: 978-1-53611-970-1 (e-book)

Caribbean Adolescents: Misuse and Abuse of Alcohol
Cecilia Hegamin-Younger and Joav Merrick (Editors)
2017. ISBN: 978-1-63485-880-9 (Hardcover)
2016. ISBN: 978-1-63485-894-6 (e-book)

Public Health: An Ecological Framework for Child Environmental Health Interventions
I. Leslie Rubin and Joav Merrick (Editors)
2017. ISBN: 978-1-53610-700-5 (Hardcover)
2017. ISBN: 978-1-53610-714-2 (e-book)

Diabetes Mellitus: A Medical History Journey
Donald E. Greydanus and Joav Merrick
2016. ISBN: 978-1-53610-094-5 (Softcover)
2016. ISBN: 978-1-53610-103-4 (e-book)

Education in Hong Kong: Service Leadership for University Students
Daniel TL Shek, Cecilia MS Ma, Li Lin and Joav Merrick (Editors)
2016. ISBN: 978-1-63484-928-9 (Hardcover)
2016. ISBN: 978-1-63484-960-9 (e-book)

Environmental Health Disparities: Costs and Benefits of Breaking the Cycle
I. Leslie Rubin and Joav Merrick (Editors)
2016. ISBN: 978-1-63484-211-2 (Hardcover)
2016. ISBN: 978-1-63484-212-9 (e-book)

Higher Education in Hong Kong: Nurturing Students to be Caring Service Leaders
Daniel TL Shek, Andrew MH Siu, Hildie Leung and Joav Merrick (Editors)
2016. ISBN: 978-1-63484-980-7 (Hardcover)
2016. ISBN: 978-1-63485-009-4 (e-book)

Measles: Epidemiology and Control of Measles in the Gweru Urban District in Zimbabwe
Tawanda Marufu, Seter Siziya, Mazyanga L. Mazaba and Joav Merrick (Editors)
2016. ISBN: 978-1-63485-559-4 (Hardcover)
2016. ISBN: 978-1-63485-573-0 (e-book)

Medical History: Some Perspectives
Donald E. Greydanus and Joav Merrick
2016. ISBN: 978-1-63484-747-6 (Hardcover)
2016. ISBN: 978-1-63484-849-7 (e-book)

Public Health: Some International Aspects
Joav Merrick (Editor)
2016. ISBN: 978-1-63484-612-7 (Hardcover)
2016. ISBN: 978-1-63484-630-1 (e-book)

Public Health: International Aspects on Environment and Health
I. Leslie Rubin and Joav Merrick (Editors)
2016. ISBN: 978-1-63484-834-3 (Hardcover)
2016. ISBN: 978-1-63484-849-7 (e-book)

Smoking and Adolescence: International Public Health Experiences
Mazyanga L. Mazaba, Seter Siziya and Joav Merrick (Editors)
2016. ISBN: 978-1-63484-311-9 (Hardcover)
2016. ISBN: 978-1-63484-312-6 (e-book)

Arbovirus: Public Health Experience from Zambia
Seter Siziya, Mazyanga L. Mazaba, and Joav Merrick (Editors)
2015. ISBN: 978-1-63463-601-8 (Hardcover)
2015. ISBN: 978-1-63463-618-6 (e-book)

Health Issues in Diverse Cultures
Cecilia Obeng, Samuel Gyasi Obeng and Joav Merrick (Editors)
2015. ISBN: 978-1-63463-613-1 (Hardcover)
2015. ISBN: 978-1-63463-619-3 (e-book)

Public Health, Social Work and Health Inequalities
Bruce D. Friedman and Joav Merrick (Editors)
2015. ISBN: 978-1-63482-838-3 (Hardcover)
2015. ISBN: 978-1-63482-850-5 (e-book)

Patient Dumping: Background, Protections, and the Mentally Ill
Tabitha E. Rivers (Editor)
2015. ISBN: 978-1-63483-726-2 (Hardcover)
2015. ISBN: 978-1-63483-727-9 (e-book)

Tomorrow's Leaders: Service Leadership and Holistic Development in Chinese University Students
Daniel TL Shek, Andrew MH Siu and Joav Merrick (Editors)
2015. ISBN: 978-1-63321-880-2 (Hardcover)
2014. ISBN: 978-1-63321-943-4 (e-book)

Environment and Public Health: Environmental Health, Law and International Perspectives
I. Leslie Rubin and Joav Merrick (Editors)
2014. ISBN: 978-1-63463-167-9 (Hardcover)
2014. ISBN: 978-1-63463-189-1 (e-book)

PUBLIC HEALTH: PRACTICES, METHODS AND POLICIES

CHILD ENVIRONMENTAL HEALTH DISPARITIES

LOOKING AT THE PRESENT AND FACING THE FUTURE

I. LESLIE RUBIN

AND

JOAV MERRICK

EDITORS

Nova Medicine & Health
New York

NOTICE TO THE READER

Library of Congress Cataloging-in-Publication Data

Names: Rubin, Isadore Leslie, editor. | Merrick, Joav, 1950- editor.
Title: Child environmental health disparities: looking at the present and facing the future / I. Leslie Rubin, Joav Merrick, editors.
Identifiers: LCCN 2020016225 (print) | LCCN 2020016226 (ebook) | ISBN 9781536178234 (hardcover) | ISBN 9781536178241 (adobe pdf)
Subjects: LCSH: Child health services--United States. | Health services accessibility--United States. | Children with social disabilities--Medical care--United States.
Classification: LCC RJ102 .C473 2020 (print) | LCC RJ102 (ebook) | DDC 362.19892--dc23
LC record available at https://lccn.loc.gov/2020016225
LC ebook record available at https://lccn.loc.gov/2020016226

Published by Nova Science Publishers, Inc. † New York

Contents

INTRODUCTION

In: Child Environmental Health Disparities ISBN: 978-1-53617-823-4
Editors: IL Rubin and J Merrick

Chapter 1

BREAK THE CYCLE OF CHILDREN'S ENVIRONMENTAL HEALTH DISPARITIES: 14TH ANNUAL REVIEW OF PROGRAM AND STUDENT PROJECTS

I Leslie Rubin[1-5,*], MD, Robert J Geller[2,3,6], MD, Claire D Coles[3,7,8], PhD, Victoria Green[3,9], MD, Abby Mutic[3,4,10], APRN, PhD, Nathan Mutic[3,4,10], Wayne Garfinkel[3,11], BSCE, Benjamin A Gitterman[12], MD and Joav Merrick[13-16], MD, MMedSci, DMSc

[1]Department of Pediatrics, Morehouse School of Medicine, Atlanta, Georgia, United States of America

---

[*] Correspondence: I Leslie Rubin, MD, Associate Professor, Department of Pediatrics, Morehouse School of Medicine, Adjunct Associate Professor, Department of Pediatrics, Emory University School of Medicine, Co-Director Southeast Pediatric Environmental Health Specialty Unit at Emory University, Founder, Break the Cycle of Health Disparities Inc Medical Director, The Rubin Center for Autism and Developmental Pediatrics. 750 Hammond Drive, Building 1, Suite 100, Atlanta, GA 30342, United States. Email lrubi01@emory.edu.

[2]Department of Pediatrics, Emory University School of Medicine, Atlanta, Georgia, United States of America
[3]Southeast Pediatric Environmental Health Specialty Unit, Emory University, Atlanta, Georgia, United States of America
[4]Break the Cycle of Health Disparities Inc, Atlanta, Georgia, United States of America
[5]The Rubin Center for Autism and Developmental Pediatrics, Atlanta, Georgia, United States of America
[6]Georgia Poison Center, Grady Health System, Atlanta, Georgia, United States of America
[7]MotherToBaby, Atlanta, Georgia, United States of America
[8]Department of Psychiatry and Behavioral Sciences and Pediatrics, Emory University School of Medicine, Atlanta, Georgia, United States of America
[9]Department of Gynecology and Obstetrics, Emory University School of Medicine, Atlanta, Georgia, United States of America
[10]Nell Hodgson Woodruff School of Nursing, Emory University, Atlanta, Georgia, United States of America
[11]Retired EPA Region 4 Children's Environmental Health Coordinator, Atlanta, Georgia, United States of America
[12]Departments of Pediatrics and Public Health, George Washington University Schools of Medicine and Public Health and Health Services, General and Community Pediatrics, Children's National Medical Center, Washington DC, United States of America
[13]National Institute of Child Health and Human Development, Jerusalem, Israel,
[14]Division of Pediatrics, Hadassah Hebrew University Medical Center, Mt Scopus Campus, Jerusalem, Israel,
[15]Kentucky Children’s Hospital, University of Kentucky College of Medicine, Lexington, Kentucky, United States of America
[16]Center for Human Development, School of Public Health, Georgia State University, Atlanta, Georgia, United States of America

ABSTRACT

Break the Cycle of Children's Environmental Health Disparities (Break the Cycle) is an annual collaborative interdisciplinary research and training program involving university students in academic tracks that focus on the impact of adverse social, economic, environmental and political factors on children's health, development, education and prospects for their future. The target populations are communities where there is a substantial measure of poverty associated with social and political marginalization predisposing to environmental degradation and risks to children's health and well-being. Each participating student is required to develop a project that focuses on preventing or reducing adverse environmental factors or their impact, in order to improve the health of the children who live in these communities. At the end of the project, students are required to present their studies and findings at a national conference and write manuscripts on their projects, which are then published in a journal supplement as well as a book. The projects cover a range of social, economic, environmental and political factors that operate over the lifespan, and have an influence on individual, family, community, and societal perspectives with an intergenerational implications. Most importantly, they add to our knowledge about children's environmental health disparities and propose solutions to reduce and eliminate health disparities and promote health equity for all children.

The papers in this publication represent the work of students who participated in the 14th Annual Break the Cycle program. The phrase 'break the cycle' in this context uses the ecological construct of the cycle of environmental health disparities, and represents a framework for projects and programs that reduce health disparities and promote health equity among children who are vulnerable as a consequence of adverse social, economic, environmental and political factors. The student projects are intended to 'break the cycle' and liberate children from the intergenerational cycle of health disparities, so they can grow and develop to their full potential. Through this academic process, the students gain knowledge, insight and skills to enable them to advance in their careers and become future leaders

INTRODUCTION

Children who grow up in poverty are more likely to be exposed to multiple adverse physical, chemical and social elements in their environment and more likely to be emotionally stressed, with multiple elements of insecurity with anxiety and fear (1). They are more likely to be exposed to poor indoor air quality, which increases the risk for asthma and respiratory disorders, and are more likely to be living in older houses with high lead levels from old paint and plumbing which can result in brain damage (2). In addition, the children are at risk for a variety of other environmental exposures, because poor neighborhoods are more likely to be located near roadways where the air is more heavily polluted with exhaust from motor vehicles, or near factories and even near toxic waste sites. Their neighborhoods and schools are often characterized by evidence of general degradation, they are more likely to be littered with trash, are poorly lit at night which increases risks of crime with fear of assault and a greater likelihood of having street drugs and drug dealers, with little to no green spaces and suitable facilities for recreation (3). Furthermore, the emotional toll on the children from multiple stressors, including food insecurity, housing insecurity, and fear of physical injury from neglect and abuse which, cumulatively can result in the physiological phenomenon of chronically elevated cortisol levels and "toxic stress" (4). The toxic stress syndrome is associated with unfavorable structural and functional changes in the brain, resulting in life-long consequences that can be associated with a reduction in brain volume in white matter, in grey matter, and specifically in the hippocampus and amygdala (5). As they reach adolescence, these children are more likely to experience school failure and engage in risky behavior, including substance abuse, gang membership, and crime which can result in incarceration or death from drugs or gun violence. The elevated cortisol levels associated with toxic stress also have a metabolic and hemodynamic impact on the cardiovascular, immune and hormonal systems, resulting in an increased likelihood of adverse health outcomes in adulthood including obesity, diabetes, and hypertension, with their associated morbidity and mortality (4).

These risks for children are greater than they are for adults, because children breathe more air, drink more water, and eat more food for their body weight than adults, so their exposure load through polluted air, water and soil is greater. Furthermore, their organs and organ systems as well as physiologic and metabolic processes are still in development, so they are more vulnerable to immediate and long term negative health outcomes (6). By the same token, the developing embryo and fetus is even more vulnerable to adverse environmental factors because the organs and organ systems are in an earlier stage of development. Therefore, the exposure of pregnant women to environmental toxins as well as emotional stress not only affect the pregnant mother's health and well-being but can also have serious and permanent effects on her fetus (7). Despite the physiological protective elements in the placenta, many toxins enter the fetal circulation and can affect organ system development, anatomically and physiologically. Many substances can cross the blood-brain barrier and adversely affect the developing brain, resulting in disorders of development and learning with risks for learning disabilities, ADHD, and even autism (8).

Children from low income and minority communities tend to live in poor neighborhoods and attend older, more dilapidated schools, with teachers who are also suffering from the stress of adverse environmental factors. Thus, the combined effects of adverse environmental and emotional stresses, along with negative educational experiences, compromise learning and even desire for learning or appreciation of the value of learning, which results in high drop-out rates and low graduation rates (9). Limited education leads to poor employment opportunities, or work with low pay, trapping the young people in the poorer neighborhoods with the older houses in states of disrepair, contributing to exposures to indoor hazards of lead, mold, and other possible contaminants, as well as emotional stress with depression, anxiety about the future with despair and social isolation (10). Those young people who drop out of school and have limited employment options with a relatively dim view of their future, may resort to drugs to feel better or crime to make money in order to live or support their habits or lifestyles. These behaviors can result in incarceration with the emotional and social consequences for the individual, the family, the community and society (11) This scenario plays out in too many cities and states in the USA and, along with draconian drug laws, has resulted in the highest incarceration rate in the world with a high percentage of young men of color in prison (12, 13). On a positive note, the statistics show that since the peak in the 1990s, the number of juvenile justice cases has decreased substantially. Although this positive trend is a result of factors beyond our personal control and reside in the hallways of local, state and federal processes, we can be encouraged to take action and strive to make a positive difference in the lives of vulnerable children, not only in reducing the negative environmental factors, but in promoting resilience through education as well as emotional and social support (14).

The assault of adverse social, economic and environmental factors on vulnerable children that results in unfavorable health, developmental, and educational outcomes, and compromises a child's opportunity for economic and social success in life, devolves into the perpetuation of an intergenerational cycle. It is the codification of this ecological construct that embodies the concept of the cycle of children's environmental health disparities (see Figure 1).

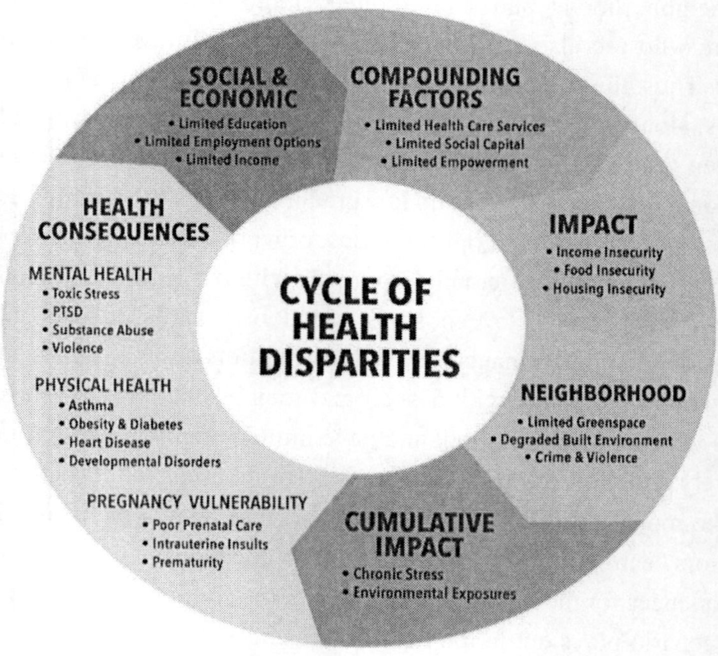

Figure 1. Cycle of environmental health disparities (15).

BREAK THE CYCLE PROGRAM

"Break the Cycle of Children's Environmental Health Disparities" (Break the Cycle) is an annual, collaborative interdisciplinary research and training program involving university students in academic tracks that focus on the impact of adverse social, economic, and environmental factors on children's health, development, and education. Each participating university student develops a project that focuses on preventing or reducing environment-related disorders for vulnerable children who live in communities where environmental hazards and emotional stresses are related to circumstances of social and economic disadvantage. At the conclusion of the project period, the students present the results of their projects at a national conference and write manuscripts on their projects which are then published in a journal supplement dedicated to the collection of projects from each given year (16). Each annual program begins with a call for proposals from a wide range of university students. The proposals are then evaluated by a competitive review process for the quality of the proposal, its relevance to children's environmental health disparities, creativity, and feasibility. The 10 best proposals are selected to work with their academic mentors and their home universities and with the Break the Cycle faculty to complete their projects. The students and their mentors are required to participate in monthly conference calls, during which the progress of each project is reviewed, additional perspectives are explored, and constructive guidance is provided. During these conference calls, the students and their mentors also have an opportunity to communicate and collaborate with their counterparts at other universities.

When the program was started, the expectation was that the projects would make a positive difference by improving the health and well-being of children, their families, and their communities. It was also envisioned that students would be inspired to pursue careers that focused on reducing health disparities and in becoming leaders for the future. Furthermore, because each student is required to have a mentor at their home university, it was anticipated that the faculty mentors would add to the literature and body of science on the subject into their curricula, and thereby promote further research and academic interest in this field (see Table 1).

Table 1. Project guidelines

• University faculty identify students who have an interest in this topic area and support the student in the selection of an idea for projects that explore environmental factors that adversely affect the health of children living in circumstances of social and economic disadvantage. Alternatively, students interested in a specific project can initiate the application process and identify mentors to work with them.
• The students submit their proposals which are reviewed by the *Break the Cycle* faculty. The process is competitive with only 10 projects being selected each year.
• During the project period, there are monthly conference calls with all students and mentors to monitor the progress of the projects, share ideas, and assure that the projects are consistent with the spirit of the *Break the Cycle* concept.
• At the end of the project period, the students present the results of their work at the annual Break the Cycle conference.
• The students are then required to write papers on their projects, which are submitted for publication in an international journal as a monograph of the *Break the Cycle* projects. The papers are also published as chapters in a book.
• The progress and careers of the participating students are tracked to evaluate the impact of their participation in the *Break the Cycle* program.

Table 2. Desired outcomes

• To inspire students from a variety of academic disciplines to explore the impact of adverse social, economic, environmental and political factors on the health, development and education of children, and to creatively generate strategies to address the challenges.
• To collaborate with an interdisciplinary team of academic leaders from a variety of different universities and colleges to get a perspective on the broader issues of this topic area
• To encourage faculty at universities who participate in this program to promote academic interest and social awareness in children's environmental health disparities
• To cultivate future leaders among the students

We also expected that the participating students would inspire peers in their academic, social and professional circles, and that the interdisciplinary nature of the program with participation of students at other universities around the world, would be stimulating and inspiring (Table 2). The 2012 survey of alumni of the program showed that the students derived significant benefit from all aspects of their participation in the process, which included the practical aspects of conducting a research project, experience in preparing and delivering a presentation and writing a manuscript. Each student gained knowledge about children's environmental health and environmental health disparities as well as being exposed to different perspectives from the other student projects (16).

Since its inception in 2004, Break the Cycle has held 14 annual programs and worked with over 120 students representing 30 different university departments in 10 states in the US, as well as students from countries in Latin America, Europe and Africa. To date, 11 monographs have been published in international journals and 11 books in a public health series. In the 2012 survey, the students rated their experience with Break the Cycle as valuable, many reporting that they pursued careers relating to their Break the cycle projects (16).

BREAK THE CYCLE 14 PROJECTS

The papers in this publication represent the interdisciplinary array of creative work by students from universities in six states in the US who participated in the 14th Annual Break the Cycle program in 2019. As usual, the papers in this volume cover a wide range of topic areas including the critical importance of maternal child relationships, adverse childhood experiences, communities, neighborhoods and gentrification, lead in drinking water, disparities in autism and systemic lupus erythematosus (SLE) diagnosis and treatment, and two new topic areas: one on the American Indian experience and the other on Medicaid coverage. While the projects on the more familiar themes add to our appreciation and understanding of the conditions addressed, the two new topic areas challenge us to think afresh about the complexity and scope of the concept of children's environmental health disparities. In addition, we identified themes across the projects, which are:

- *Cost of care.* Healthcare financing is a critical factor in assuring access to quality diagnostic and therapeutic services. This is the focus of the student project in this series on expansion of Medicaid services and health outcomes, but it also has relevance across other projects, such as access to services for children with autism. There is no question that Medicaid has improved access to healthcare for vulnerable populations in our society, particularly for children from low income families, but there remains room for improvement at a systemic level.
- *Literacy and health literacy.* The importance of speech, language, communication, and understanding of the spoken and written word in health and healthcare is essential. The projects that address this topic area range from the importance of infants being exposed to complex speech and learning vocabulary early in life, to the importance of health literacy of mothers in taking care of their infants, to teenagers with SLE being able to read and interpret the doses of their medication. Ultimately, this speaks to the importance of a good general education as well as being educated about wellness and maintaining good health.
- *Neighborhoods, communities and culture.* Our neighborhoods and the communities are the building blocks of our society. Projects in this series examine the specific communities of American Indian pregnant women and the young mothers of infants from Paraguay, which effectively opened the conversation to exploring cultural identity and how to effect positive change without losing sight of the respect for the importance of cultural history and cultural ties and how these affect health literacy and healthy practices. In addition, there are the African American communities in North Carolina which are geographically isolated from municipal water resources and must rely on well-water which is more likely to be contaminated. Then there are the low-income communities living in degraded neighborhoods which are undergoing transition to an upgraded and more upscale built environment. As a consequence, families in the old neighborhoods are required to adapt to the

changing environment and demographics or forced to relocate; either way there is disruption of their communities with adverse social and emotional consequences.

- *Individual vs population or statistics*. The values of science and its practical translation for use in real life are critical to our understanding of ourselves, the environment, and our interaction with the environment. While statistics are the foundational basis of our science today, the appreciation of the findings may not be readily apparent in real life. In several of the papers in this series, most notably in the two on autism disparities and the work on the mothers in Paraguay, there are vignettes of what some of the subjects reported of their experiences. These vignettes help to breathe life into the science and help in conveying an understanding of the findings and their implications.

The following are brief reviews of the Break the Cycle 14 student projects in this volume.

The development of a prenatal care health literacy instrument for American Indian mothers

This project is the first in the 14 years of Break the Cycle to focus on the American Indian community. As of 2017, there were an estimated 5.6 million people who were classified as American Indian and Alaska Native comprising 1.7 percent of the total US population (17). American Indians were on American continents for millennia before the European conquerors arrived and decimated the large Native American population with unfamiliar diseases, and with sophisticated weaponry and strategies honed from the frequent and often protracted battles and wars fought on European and Asian soil. After countless battles and wars between the European settlers and the Native Americans, so-called treaties partitioned American Indian land into fragments for each of the remaining tribal groups scattered across the continent, disconnected from one another. This disconnection had some basis in the different identities and cultures of the extant tribes at that time and may have seemed logical, but the dispersion and local tribal affiliations has precluded a cohesive and compelling coalition that, theoretically could, by virtue of a unified voice, become a force to be reckoned with, politically and economically. Furthermore, the conquering armies and immigrant people exerted power over the indigenous population through subjugation with systematic and determined disruption and destruction of the existing cultural norms, languages, practices and beliefs, and through the imposition of the conquerors' culture, language, customs and beliefs.

Consequently, the people who once proudly and powerfully populated and dominated the American continents, effectively became and, even in the 21st Century, remain second class citizens. In the US, they have become a relatively forgotten and neglected people. Apart from the imagery and pageantry, American Indian communities remain in remote and disconnected parcels of land, in situations of social, economic and political isolation. As a result, unemployment, poverty and despair result in the ills of the people and their society, effectively trapped in the cycle of environmental health disparities (17, 18). However, despite the prevailing poverty, lack of good education and healthcare services, high unemployment, as well as other adverse economic and social factors, there are positive trends with modest individual and group successes. In his book on the resilience of the American Indian Community, David Treuer reviews and revises the history of the people as has been told over time to the present, and builds a picture of a proud and resilient group of people who have survived the genocide and are rebuilding their identity and defining their role on the global stage (19).

There is much work to be done to improve the situation for most people of Native American heritage and to rebuild their communities, their educational institutions, and the provision of healthcare, especially for the children. To this end, the United States Centers for Disease Control and Prevention (CDC) is working with relevant agencies to foster cooperation and promote good health (20).

In her project, Jordyn Gunville, MPH, from the Center for American Indian Community Health, Department of Family Medicine, at the

University of Kansas Medical Center, focused on the high infant mortality rate among the American Indian population, which is nearly four times that for white infants. She examined the role of education and health literacy in promoting a healthy attitude towards pregnancy and prenatal care in not only reducing infant mortality, but also in cultivating a healthier approach to childbearing and childrearing. She makes a very persuasive argument that a focus on literacy and health literacy are crucial to improving awareness of health for the mother, for the child and for the community and for the society at large. The long-term outlook for this approach lies in a positive trans-generational impetus to improved health, improved education, and improved family, community, and societal stability. The next step in the process is to develop strategies to raise awareness in promoting policies and implement practices that will reduce infant mortality and measurably improve child health and education. This student has demonstrated that promoting literacy and health literacy brings substantial benefit in the promise of breaking the cycle of health disparities, particularly for this population.

Barriers and opportunities for young caregivers to provide nurturing care in low income communities in Paraguay

Although we have previously had student projects from Central and South American countries, including Chile, Mexico and Brazil, this is the first from Paraguay. The population profiles of each of the Latin American countries is unique, yet there are themes and patterns common to all (21). Prior to the European invasion, as in North America, the lands were populated by native tribes, communities with political and economic powers, including great civilizations and empires. The European settlers and conquistadors overpowered and overwhelmed the local peoples with wars, and subjugated them with oppressive policies. At times, there were conflicts and even battles and wars between neighboring countries. Over time, each of the Latin American countries has undergone political changes and upheavals as well as political convulsions and revolutions, cycling through various forms of government, including dictatorships, until eventually settling, for the most part in the 21st century, into relative democracies. The reality in many Latin American Countries is the wide gap between the rich and the poor as measured by the Gini index (22), which is an international measure of economic inequality in a particular country. The lower the score, the more equitable the income distribution. Few regions in the world are as unequal as Latin America (23). Out of the 20 countries worldwide when measuring high income inequality on the Gini Index, eight are Latin American while the rest are in Sub-Saharan Africa. On a positive note, Latin America is a region to have made the most progress in attenuating wage inequality since the turn of the century, lowering its Gini index by 6 points from 2002 to 2013.

In her project, Jimena Vallejos MPA, studying at Columbia University School of International and Public Affairs in New York, focused on early childhood development and examined child rearing practices in poor neighborhoods in Paraguay using the WHO/UNICEF/World Bank document entitled Nurturing Care for Early Childhood Development: A Framework for Helping Children Survive and Thrive to Transform Health and Human Potential (24). In her project, she interviewed families and catalogued their knowledge, child rearing practices, and the challenges they face.

She also listed the various agencies and policies that have been developed in response to the situation in Paraguay, and made some specific recommendations of her own, most importantly to focus on the families, strengthen the services, monitor progress and keep track with data to validate the outcomes. This is another strong example of a student project making a difference and offering practical strategies to break the cycle.

Breaking the Cycle of childhood adversity through pediatric primary care screening and interventions: A pilot study

Although the association between chronic disorders and illnesses in adults with early childhood traumas has been documented, it was not until a large study of almost 10,000 subjects from a large health maintenance organization (HMO) in collaboration with the Centers for Disease Control and Prevention (CDC) was published in 1998, that the codification of Adverse Childhood Experiences (ACEs) was clearly linked to adverse health outcomes in adulthood (25).

This study linked a set of 10 ACEs in childhood categorized as reflecting abuse, neglect or household dysfunction and characterized as physical, emotion and sexual abuse or physical and emotional neglect; household dysfunction include mental illness, substance abuse, domestic violence, family disruption, or a family member who is incarcerated. The physical and physiological adverse health outcomes they identified were, metabolic disorders such as obesity and diabetes, cardiac disorders and stroke, chronic lung disease, as well as increased likelihood of broken bones and cancer, all reducing life expectancy. They also had an increased likelihood of patterns of substance abuse, with addictions to tobacco, alcohol, eating, sex, and to drugs such as opioids, all with consequent risks of early death. They also identified a greater likelihood of depression with increased risk for suicide attempts and successes. Furthermore, the patterns of mental and physical disorders make it less likely that they would hold a steady job, resulting in reduced income and increased likelihood of dependence on public welfare. In all, not only did ACEs lead to adverse health, behavioral and social outcomes aggravating the stress on the individual and family, but also on the community and society at large.

Furthermore, the study found a positive correlation between the number of ACEs and the number and severity of adverse health outcomes, especially with those who experienced four or more ACEs compared to those who had experienced none. For example, they found 4- to 12-fold increased risk for alcoholism, drug abuse, depression, and suicide attempt; a 2-to 4-fold increases in smoking, poor self-rated health, having more than 50 sexual intercourse partners, and sexually transmitted disease; as well as a 1.4- to 1.6-fold increase in physical inactivity and severe obesity. The intergenerational consequences are likewise profoundly disturbing – see the cycle of health disparities (see Figure 1).

At the 12th annual Break the Cycle program, there was a symposium on resilience during which one of the presenters, a woman who had a high childhood ACEs score, spoke about her childhood and resultant physical, emotional and social disorders of her adulthood, and how she overcame them to find a job at the CDC working the field of ACEs (14). The lessons from her life story illustrate how people can overcome ACEs and develop resilience to become successful, functioning and healthy adults.

Importantly, the project by Cristian Quizhpi, MD, a pediatric resident in the Department of Pediatrics at East Tennessee State University, looks at how ACEs and their consequences can be identified at an early age through screening and intervention in primary care pediatric settings and strategies can be developed to increase the likelihood that the children being seen in infancy and childhood will escape ACEs and grow up will become healthy, competent, functioning and independent adults who make positive contributions to society.

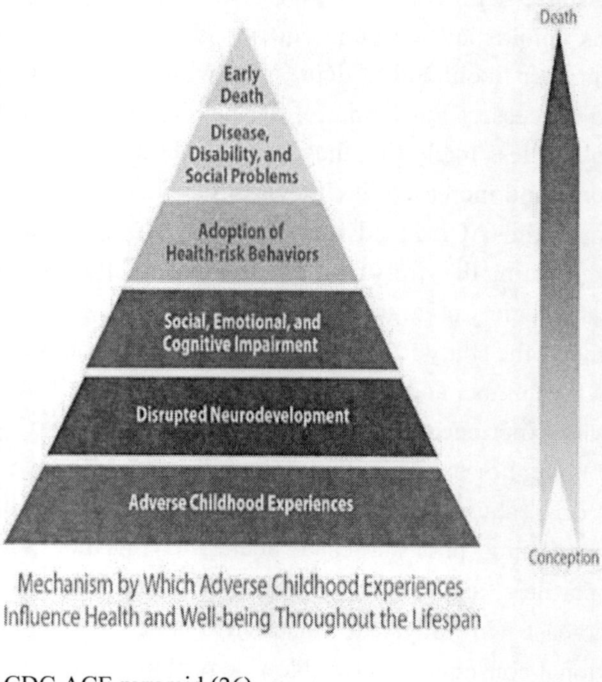

Figure 2. The CDC ACE pyramid (26).

Educating clinic stakeholders to enhance early learning environments through pediatric well-child visits

The human brain enables sophisticated levels of cognitive and intellectual function, especially with communication and socialization. Most of brain development in the proliferation of numbers of cells, in migration of neurons to their place in the cerebral cortex and with the formation of a network of connections between the neurons, occurs before birth. After birth, the major factor in brain development is in the myelination process, which contributes to brain growth in size as well as physiologically enhancing the speed of neural transmissions facilitating thinking processes and helping to provide the increasing physical, cognitive and social abilities that will serve as a basis for independent functional and social living. The next critical element in brain growth and development is in utilizing the infrastructural elements of the brain in the process of building competence, confidence and independence through enhancing neural connections and networks. While much of the brain development is genetically determined, there are powerful environmental forces at play, prenatally as well as postnatally, that influence all aspects of brain development, especially in the development of neuronal connections directly or indirectly through epigenetic mechanisms (27).

It is during these first three critical years of brain development when environmental factors play the largest role in brain development in positive as well as negative ways. Just as adverse childhood experiences have a profound negative effect on brain structure and function, positive influences such as maternal-infant bonding, intense mother-child interaction, parental communication around the child and with the child, and reading to the child frequently, have a positive effect on the child though the positive effect on brain function, resulting in greater chances of maturation, independence and success in life (28).

In their project, Cori Walker, a medical student at the University of Chicago, and Asher Liu, a high school student, partnered to raise awareness in pediatric offices of the importance of promoting parent-child interaction towards improving the child's experience of language and promote enhanced language development. This project was supported in part by the

Thirty Million Words (TMW) program, which has as its premise that children from high income families will hear 45 million words by three years of age, while the three year-old of a low income or welfare family will only hear about 13 million words, a gap of about 30 million words (29). The goal of the TMW program is to reduce that gap, and the project by these two students demonstrated that a primary care pediatric office is a good place to start, with the encouragement of stimulation of infant speech development. Similar programs like "Reach Out and Read" also focus on primary care pediatric offices to promote reading among low income children (30). Each effort at increasing literacy for children, in encouraging children to read and communicate effectively, plays a part in increasing the promise of success in life, thereby contributing towards breaking the cycle of children's environmental health disparities.

Engaging parents of children with autism spectrum disorder to identify urban and rural health disparities and factors related to delayed diagnosis and treatment and autism disparities: Structural and institutional barriers

Autism spectrum disorder (ASD) is the current term used to diagnose children who have a neurodevelopmental disorder characterized by delays and unusual patterns of speech and language development, and unusual patterns of communication interaction and socialization, along with a need for sameness, with obsessions or repetitive behaviors. An ASD diagnosis manifests in a large range of differences in complexity and severity of the symptoms – hence the use of word "spectrum" in the diagnostic label.

The diagnosis has evolved since the first description in 1943 by Leo Kanner (1894-1981) of infantile autism (31), then, over decades, the less dramatic expressions became characterized as pervasive developmental disorder of childhood, through the inclusion of Asperger syndrome describing children who were verbal and intelligent, sometimes extraordinarily intelligent, often with a singular focus of interest. Interestingly, Hans Asperger (1906-1980) wrote his paper in 1944 (32), but because it was written in German, it only came to clinical attention in the USA after it had been translated into English in the late 1980s (33). Over the course of the decades since the original description by Kanner in 1943, almost 80 years ago, the number of children who have been diagnosed has grown from one 1 in 10,000 in the early decades to 1 in 150 in the CDC report of 2002, to 1 in 59 in the CDC report of 2018 (34). Part of the increase in prevalence is certainly the expansion of the diagnostic umbrella, but there may well be a real increase in prevalence, likely related to genetic and epigenetic factors precipitated by the profusion of chemicals in our environment (35, 36). Be that as it may, it is critically important to make an early diagnosis and institute therapy as soon as possible, to improve functional outcome and reduce complications (37).

Two student projects this year looked at disparities for children with ASD with delays in diagnosis and limited initiation of therapy related to type of insurance coverage and to geographic location. Alice Hong, a student at Georgia Institute of Technology, School of History and Sociology in Atlanta, Georgia, looked at low-income minority families, often in a single parent household, on public health insurance. Amy Blumling, a student at Emory University Nell Hodgson Woodruff School of Nursing, looked at low income rural populations. In both cases, there were delays in diagnosis and difficulty in accessing necessary services. In both projects, students' methodology reviewed the demographics and other characteristics, but explored individual circumstances of the families, providing not only the statistical information on the situation but delving into the personal and real-life challenges and emotions, as well as coping styles of the families. Both provided a rich insight into the lives of these two groups of families and communities and generated a sympathetic set of recommendations and strategies to reduce these disparities. Since the situation is not uncommon in lower income, often minority, families, a Break the Cycle of Autism Disparities Program was started, which promises a systemic look at how to improve the access to timely diagnosis and appropriate therapies (38).

Water infrastructure and childhood blood lead levels: characterizing the effects of exclusion from municipal services in Wake County, North Carolina, USA

Water is an essential part of life and access to clean drinking water is at the core of the Sustainable Development Goal #6 of "clean accessible water for all." A driving force of the goal is a call for "increased investment in management of freshwater ecosystems and sanitation facilities on a local level in several developing countries" (39). In the US, there is substantial pollution of many bodies of water, most notably in the Great Lakes, which was, in the early 1970's, the impetus for the Clean Water Act (40).

Allison C Clonch, a Public Health student at the Gillings School of Global Public Health at the University of North Carolina, Chapel Hill, demonstrated the presence of increased lead in well water in poor African American neighborhoods in North Carolina. Lead is toxic to children and often causes brain damage, placing the children at a disadvantage academically and socially thereby contributing to the cycle of environmental health disparities (41). The families in these communities use well water because their districts have been excluded from municipal water supply. This is the 2nd project from this academic center looking at the impact of this discriminatory practice in not providing municipal water to a community, thereby putting children at significant risk for the immediate and long-term adverse health outcomes of lower quality than that of the municipal water (42). Raising awareness of this situation is the first step in breaking the cycle. The next step is to change the situation by restructuring the water supply. The student appropriately asks for "more regulatory oversight and water quality tests of private water systems or facilitating access to municipal supplies in order to mitigate the impacts associated with childhood lead exposure."

Self-reported neighborhood quality and children's depression symptoms in a gentrifying Northern Manhattan

Gentrification refers to the process of change taking place in an older, low income, often minority and most-likely degraded neighborhood, when relatively wealthier residents and businesses move into the neighborhood because of the lower rent and opportunity to build, restructure and grow (43). The initial influx is gradual but over the course of time, the trickle becomes a flow and at some point, the neighborhood is transformed from the old, often dilapidated and neglected character, to a modern, often creative one, with desirable amenities such as restaurants and boutiques that attract new, more affluent residents and visitors. Often a large chain business will anchor in the neighborhood, offering the local residents access to more amenities and products with further income generation for the area making it more affluent and desirable for the residents. For those moving into the neighborhoods it is exciting and promising, and for the business it can be lucrative, but for the long-term residents for whom the neighborhood has long been home, and the community a source of support and identity, the change may not be positive and can be disruptive.

The anthropologic history of cities and neighborhoods is one of flux. Cities were often established based on access to transportation routes, or near a sizable waterway for water supply and transportation. As cities grew and flourished, they often became overcrowded and required some strategy to deal with the growth. In the US, as in other parts of the world, the arrival of the automobile altered the patterns of urban living dramatically. When transportation was limited to pedestrian or horse driven vehicles, proximity to the necessities of day-to-day life was a critical determinant of residential location. However, with the advent and increasing availability of the automobile, proximity became less important because people could live some distance from the city and drive to work. Thus, began the suburbanization of society. The migration of people with financial means to purchase homes and cars to the suburbs led to dramatic suburban growth. The resulting vacant urban residential areas provided an opportunity for people of lower income to settle and find work for themselves, schools for their children, and communities of people like themselves to provide the social and emotional support necessary for health and stability (44). Unfortunately, over time, inner cities became concentrated with low income families and communities, while their more affluent counterparts were living in the suburbs. This situation became informally institutionalized, if not codified and calcified over the course of the early second half of the 20th century (45). Then, towards the end of the 20th Century, for a variety of social and economic factors, younger people with means began to move back to the cities and started the trend of gentrification, which continues today in many large cities in the US (43).

In her project, Teresa Durham, at the Columbia Center for Children's Environmental Health, Columbia University in New York City, examined the impact on the health and well-being of children in the rapidly gentrifying neighborhoods in Northern Manhattan. The Columbia Center has been working in this neighborhood for many years, tracking the children and families, and has collected data on the impact of gentrification on the community in Northern Manhattan, which their students are now mining. A prior student from the Center who had participated in the Break the Cycle program looked at the impact on children's health focusing on children's nutritional status (46). In her work, Ms. Dunham focused on the mental health of the children, particularly anxiety and depression. She found that although anxiety was a common symptom, it was not greater than the baseline level of anxiety of children in the neighborhood under stress. She did, however, find a level of depression greater than baseline among the children. Of interest, her results revealed that the children who exhibited the symptoms of depression were those whose mothers rated their total neighborhood quality as being more stressful over a six-year time period than the children of mothers who reported their neighborhood to be less stressful. This study helps us to recognize the importance of understanding the experience of stress and its manifestation in anxiety and depression in children, and the management of stress as important in promoting health for the children. It is also helpful in determining interventions for the children and their families when a neighborhood is undergoing such dramatic upheaval and the anticipation of a possible move from the familiar and comfortable home and neighborhood environment, to an unknown destination. The question to be asked is whether the measure of stress reported by some of the mothers was a valid reflection of overall neighborhood stress, or the stress was personal and was associated with other factors within the family in terms of coping mechanisms and resilience, which could then affect her children. In addition, communities must consider their collective and individual responsibilities to be aware of the impact of gentrification on children's health and development and to help prevent the inevitable associated health impacts, such as anxiety and depression (47).

The impact of childhood exercise and socioeconomic status on coping strategies and resilience in college students

It is well recognized that children from lower socioeconomic circumstances are less likely to attend college and, if they do, they are less likely to graduate and less likely to attend a post-secondary school of higher education. The statistics are difficult to refute and extremely sobering – see the Figure 3 below (48).

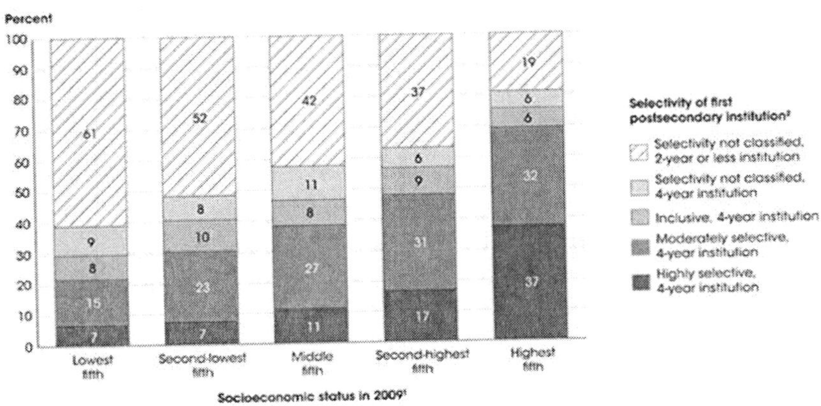

Figure 3. Among 2009 ninth-graders who had enrolled in postsecondary education by 2016, percentage distribution of selectivity of students' first postsecondary institution, by socioeconomic status (48).

Among several reasons given for this phenomenon, one pragmatic reason is that primary education is not as effective or at a level of similar quality in poorer neighborhoods, where the children and their families have less financial resources and the children may need to work to sustain income and pay for college. Other reasons relate to a 'sense of self' or self-esteem and appreciation of one's capability and potential.

In her project, Leah Postilnik, BSN, a student at the College of Nursing, University of Massachusetts, examined the role of exercise and physical activity as a factor in shaping resilience in those students from communities of lower socioeconomic status (SES). Although there are fewer students from lower SES communities who attend college, and, of those who do attend, a significant number who do not complete their courses, there are students with a background of low-SES who do attend college and university and who do thrive and succeed. Students from low-SES background who do succeed do so because of an ability to overcome adversity through resilience. The factors that determine resilience may be genetic and inherent in the personality of the individual, but include environmental and experiential elements as well, most significantly is the presence in their lives of a caring, supportive encouraging, and committed adult, be it a parent, grandparent, other relative, teacher or parent figure in their communities (14). In addition, social networks of support, positive role models, a good education, intellectual stimulation, self-discipline and positive, physical exercise also contribute significantly to the development of resilience. Ms. Postilnik examined the role of exercise in promoting and reflecting resilience and academic achievement, and found a positive correlation between resilience and exercise frequency. When controlling for other variables, college exercise was the only variable shown to predict resilience, and middle school exercise predicted high school and college exercise. Implications of these results suggest the need for interventions to increase exercise for children from low SES environments, establish exercise habits early in childhood, and use exercise as a tool to promote resilience. Exercise may not be the sole factor, but is a strong and positive force in promoting physical, mental, emotional and social health, which in turn promotes self-esteem and a positive approach to life and its challenges and break the cycle of health disparities.

Health literacy in pediatric onset lupus erythematosus

Systemic lupus erythematosus (SLE) is a complex autoimmune disorder. It can affect many organ systems in the body as well as the brain, manifesting in psychiatric disorders. In more severe expressions of the condition, it can result in organ system failure, particularly renal. In all, SLE causes much physical and mental suffering and can shorten life expectancy. Because it affects many organ systems, the person with SLE is likely to need the expertise of a variety of different medical specialists as well as therapists and more often than not, require multiple medications.

This lifestyle of multiple physician and therapy visits, that consume significant hours in any day in travel and waiting in addition to the specific clinic visits, can be physically and emotionally stressful and draining of energy and time for education, recreation and socialization. The combination of the impact of the disease process and the stresses associated with the condition and its management, compound the situation. On a positive note, much research has been done to understand and manage the condition, reducing the likelihood of complications and mitigating severity. Further, in recognition of the need for close monitoring of the condition and continuity of care, multidisciplinary clinics and centers have been established where people with lupus can go to get their necessary practical help and suppoert that is configured to provide comprehensive, coordinated care to people with lupus, to monitor their progress, assure optimal care, and deliver as good physical, emotional and social health outcomes as possible for each individual.

Catherine Park, MD, a Fellow in the Department of Pediatrics, Division of Nephrology at Emory University School of Medicine, where she serves children with lupus, compared the clinical profiles of children from poor circumstances to those from more affluent backgrounds, and found that the poorer children were more likely to be diagnosed later than their more affluent counterparts, were more likely to be exposed to second hand tobacco smoke (which is known to aggravate the clinical condition), and tended to have more serious complications with more emergency department visits. She administered health literacy tests to the children, and found that the children from the low SES group had lower numeracy literacy than their more affluent counterparts. She postulated that the lower numeracy literacy possibly contributed to their increased rate of medical complications, because of their limited ability to accurately read the instructions on their often multiple bottles of medication, as well as to read the details on food labels. Although her sample size was small, the findings were significant, and reflect the importance of literacy and health literacy. In addition, this speaks to the critical importance of a good education for children, particularly for children from low SES background, with emphasis on fundamental skills such as reading and math, which better prepares them for life and its challenges, and helps them lead healthier lives and break the cycle of health disparities.

Although it is not addressed in this paper, the issue of cost of care and insurance reimbursement with Medicaid is a significant factor in the care of SLE. The condition is often complex and requires frequent, and expensive, specialized medical attention, with multiple medications and increase in emergency department visits, not to mention the incidental costs of transportation and lost hours at school or work for parents. While these costs may be reasonably borne by more affluent families with private health insurance, they are more likely to be burdensome for lower SES families and may seriously affect their livelihood. Fortunately, there is a safety net in publicly funded medical insurance through Medicaid, which helps to secure the necessary medical care, but not necessarily the incidental and collateral costs.

Did Medicaid expansion decrease disparities for receipt of preventive medical care among vulnerable children?

In 14 years of Break the Cycle programs, this is the first student project that examines children's health insurance as a factor in breaking the cycle of children's environmental health disparities. In US society, where access to health care is dependent on the cost of health care and reimbursement to the providers of healthcare, the ability of a family to pay for the care becomes a powerful determinant in access to, and provision of healthcare, be it episodic, routine or long term. In the US, private health insurance is a critical resource to secure necessary healthcare. Families who can afford the cost of insurance premiums have relatively easier access to quality healthcare. For low income families who do not receive assistance in covering the cost of health insurance premiums, there is Medicaid. Medicaid in the US is a federal and state program that helps cover medical costs for some people with limited income and resources.

The history of American society and government in developing and providing public health insurance through Medicaid, has evolved over the past half century from the establishment of health insurance for the elderly though Medicare established in 1965, based as a policy framework on the social Security Act of 1935. Over the decades, the benefits have been extended to an increasing list of vulnerable populations through the Home and Community Based Services (HCBS) Medicaid waiver programs, and more recently, the Children's Health Insurance Program (CHIP). The most recent evolutionary component of the Medicaid program has been the Affordable Care Act (ACA) of 2010, which expanded the services further (see Figure 4 for details on the evolution of Medicaid services). Of note is that the Medicaid program is a Federal-State partnership, and not all states in the US opted into the ACA.

In her project on whether Medicaid expansion resulted in improved healthcare to vulnerable children, Patricia Daniel, PhD, from the Center for Leadership in Disability, at Georgia State University in Atlanta, Georgia, compared data from those states that opted into the ACA and those that did not. Data suggest that Medicaid does contribute to improvement in health of the populations it serves, and Dr. Daniel was able to demonstrate this in her study. At the time of this writing, national political debate is examining the pros and cons of further Medicaid expansion, with some suggesting a universal coverage model similar to a number of Western European nations and Canada or complete abandonment of the ACA. Whatever the outcome of the debate, the important fact is that Medicaid covers one in five people in the US and is the main sources of coverage and access to healthcare for vulnerable populations. This is especially true for children, the elderly population, people with disabilities, as well as people with low or no income, who cannot afford private insurance; as such, it has been and continues to be of great benefit not only to the individuals and families served, but also to society at large (49).

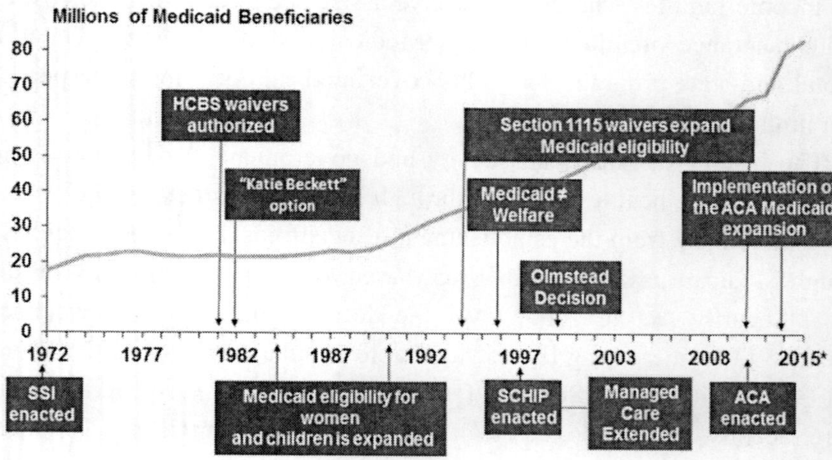

Figure 4. Medicaid has evolved over time 1972-2015 (49).

Conclusion

As with our previous Break the Cycle programs, each student had identified a different component of the Cycle of Children's Environmental Health Disparities and highlighted the way in which the cycle can be broken at that point and the health of vulnerable children can be improved. In the process, the students benefited from creatively developing a project, translating it into action, performing the research, presenting the results of their projects at a national conference and now writing manuscripts for publication in this publication. In addition, their mentors, as well as their peers and we, the Break the Cycle Faculty, have also learned and benefitted from this collective experience. Furthermore, our society gains by their work in the present, and will undoubtedly gain in the future when this cohort of students become our leaders.

ACKNOWLEDGMENTS

Thanks to the additional editors of some of the papers who have given of their time and expertise, much appreciated especially our trusted friend and editor David Ervin, as well as Erin Lebow-Skelly. This publication was supported by the cooperative agreement award number 5 NU61TS000237-05 from the Agency for Toxic Substances and Disease Registry (ATSDR). Its contents are the responsibility of the authors and do not necessarily represent the official views of the Agency for Toxic Substances and Disease Registry (ATSDR). The U.S. Environmental Protection Agency (EPA) supports the PEHSU by providing partial funding to ATSDR under Inter-Agency Agreement number DW-75-95877701. Neither EPA nor ATSDR endorse the purchase of any commercial products or services mentioned in PEHSU publications.

REFERENCES

[1] Hodgkinson S, Godoy L, Beers LS, Lewin A. Improving mental health access for low-income children and families in the primary care setting. Pediatrics 2017;139(1):e20151175.

[2] Adamkiewicz G, Zota AR, Fabian MP, Chahine T, Julien R, Spengler JD, Levy JI. Moving environmental justice indoors: Understanding structural influences on residential exposure patterns in low-income communities. Am J Public Health 2011;101(suppl 1):S238–45.

[3] Hood E. Dwelling disparities: How poor housing leads to poor health. Environ Health Perspect 2005;113(5):A310–7. doi: 10.1289/ehp.113-a310.

[4] Shonkoff JP, Garner AS, Committee on Psychosocial Aspects of Child and Family Health, Committee on Early Childhood, Adoption, and Dependent Care, Section on Developmental and Behavioral Pediatrics. The lifelong effects of early childhood

adversity and toxic stress. Pediatrics 2012;129(1):e232-46. doi: 10.1542/peds.2011-2663. Epub 2011 Dec 26.

[5] Luby J, Belden A, Botteron K, Marrus N, Harms MP, Babb C, et al. The effects of poverty on childhood brain development: The mediating effect of caregiving and stressful life. JAMA Pediatr 2013;167(12):1135-42.

[6] Children's unique vulnerabilities to environmental hazards In: Etzel RA, Balk SJ, eds. Pediatric environmental health, 4th edition: Itasca IL; American Academy of Pediatrics, 2019:17-31.

[7] Toxic or environmental preconceptual and prenatal exposures. In: Etzel RA, Balk, SJ, eds. Pediatric environmental health, 4th edition: Itasca IL; American Academy of Pediatrics, 2019:101-18.

[8] Rubin IL. Fetal environment and risks for intellectual and developmental disabilities. In: Rubin IL, Merrick J, Greydanus DE, Patel DR, eds. Health care for people with intellectual and developmental disabilities across the lifespan. Cham, Switzerland: Springer, 2016:363-70.

[9] Wodtke GT, Elwert F, Harding DJ. Poor families, poor neighborhoods: How family poverty intensifies the impact of concentrated disadvantage on high school graduation. Ann Arbor, MI: University of Michigan Population Studies Center Research Report 2012:12-776.

[10] Mood C, Jonsson JO. The social consequences of poverty: An empirical test on longitudinal data. Soc Indic Res 2016;127:633–52. doi: 10.1007/s11205-015-0983-9.

[11] Rubin IL, Geller RJ, Martinuzzi K, Howett M, Gitterman BA, Wells LM, Garfinkel W, Coles CD, Merrick J. Children's environmental health disparities: The costs and benefits of breaking the cycle. Int J Child Health Hum Dev 2016;9(4):419-30.

[12] The Sentencing Project fact sheet. Trends in US corrections. URL: https://www.sentencingproject.org/wp-content/uploads/2016/01/Trends-in-US-Corrections.pdf.

[13] Sickmund M, Sladky TJ, Kang W, Puzzanchera C. Easy access to the census of juveniles in residential placement, 2016. URL: http://www.ojjdp.gov/ojstatbb/ezacjrp.

[14] Rubin IL. Resilience: A commentary on breaking the cycle. Int Public Health J 2018;10(3):247-64.

[15] Rubin IL, Geller RJ, Martinuzzi K, Howett M, Gitterman BA, Wells L, et al. Break the cycle of children's environmental health disparities: An ecological framework. Int Public Health J 2017;9(2):115-249.

[16] Rubin IL, Oves D, Nodvin J, Geller RJ, Howett M, Martinuzzi K, et al. The learning experience of 'Break the cycle' program: Survey of past students. In: Rubin IL, Merrick J, eds. Environmental health disparities. New York: Nova Science, 2016:171-85.

[17] US Department of Health and Human Services, Office of Minority Health. Profile: American Indian/Alaska Native. URL: https://www.minorityhealth.hhs.gov/omh/browse.aspx?lvl=3&lvlid=62.

[18] Sarche M, Spicer P. Poverty and health disparities for American Indian and Alaska Native children: Current knowledge and future prospects. Ann NY Acad Sci 2008;1136:126-36. doi: 10.1196/annals.1425.017.

[19] Treuer D. The heartbeat of Wounded Knee: Native America from 1890 to the present. New York: Penguin Random House, 2019.

[20] CDC Tribal Health. URL: https://www.cdc.gov/tribal/index.html.

[21] LatinoStories.com. US Department of State Histories of Latin American Countries. URL: http://latinostories.com/Latin_America_Resources/Latin_American_History_Profiles/History_of_Latin_American_Countries.htm.

[22] The World Bank. GINI level. URL: https://data.worldbank.org/indicator/SI.POV.GINI.

[23] Americas Society. Council on the Americas. Weekly Chart: Income inequality in Latin America. URL: https://www.as-coa.org/articles/weekly-chart-income-inequality-latin-america.

[24] Nurturing care for early childhood development: A framework for helping children survive and thrive to transform health and human potential. Geneva: World Health Organization, 2018.

[25] Felitti VJ, Anda RF, Nordenberg D, Williamson DF, Spitz AM, Edwards V, et al. Relationship of childhood abuse and household dysfunction to many of the leading causes of death in adults. The Adverse Childhood Experiences (ACE) study. Am J Prev Med 1998;14(4):245–58.

[26] CDC Violence Prevention. About the CDC-Kaiser ACE Study. URL: https://www.cdc.gov/violenceprevention/childabuseandneglect/acestudy/about.html.

[27] Gilmore JH, Knickmeyer RC, Gao W Imaging structural and functional brain development in early childhood. Nat Rev Neurosci 2018;19(3):123- 37. doi: 10.1038/nrn.2018.1.

[28] Miguel PM, Pereira LO, Silveira PP, Meaney MJ. Early environmental influences on the development of children's brain structure and function. Dev Med Child Neurol 2019;61(10):1127-33. doi: 10.1111/dmcn.14182.

[29] Suskind D, Leung C, Zimowski M, Hernandez M. A new clinical tool to access parental expectations and knowledge about child cognitive and language development: The SPEAK. Pediatrics 2018;142 (1 MeetingAbstract):775. URL: https://doi.org/10.1542/peds.142.1_MeetingAbstract.775.

[30] Thakur K, Sudhanthar S, Sigal Y, Mattarella N. Improving early childhood literacy and school readiness through Reach Out and Read (ROR) program. BMJ Qual Improv Rep 2016;5(1):pii:u209772.w4137. doi: 10.1136/bmjquality.u209772.w4137.

[31] Kanner L. Autistic disturbances of affective contact. Nerv Child 1943;2:217–50.

[32] Asperger H. [Die 'Autistischen psychopathen' im kindesalter]. Arch Psychiatr Nervenkr 1944;117:76–136.

[33] Wing L. Reflections on opening Pandora's box. J Autism Dev Disord 2005;35(2):197-203.

[34] Baio J, Wiggins L, Christensen DL, Maenner MJ, Daniels J, Warren Z, al. Prevalence of autism spectrum disorder among children aged 8 years: Autism and Developmental Disabilities Monitoring Network, 11 Sites, United States, 2014. MMWR 2018;67(6):1–23. doi: http://dx.doi.org/10.15585/mmwr.ss6706a1external icon.

[35] Ye BS, Leung AOW, Wong MH. The association of environmental toxicants and autism spectrum disorders in children. Environ Pollut 2017;227:234242. doi: 10.1016/j.envpol.2017.04.039.

[36] Pelch KE, Bolden AL, Kwiatkowski CF. Environmental chemicals and autism: A scoping review of the human and animal research. Environ Health Perspect 2019;127(4):46001. doi: 10.1289/EHP4386.

[37] Elder JH, Kreider CM, Brasher SN, Ansell M. Clinical impact of early diagnosis of autism on the prognosis and parent–child relationships. Psychol Res Behav Manag 2017;10:283–92. doi: 10.2147/PRBM.S117499.

[38] Break the Cycle of autism disparities. URL: https://www.breakthecycleprogram.org/break-the-cycle-of-autism.

[39] UN Sustainable Development Goals. Goal 6: Ensure access to water and sanitation for all. URL: https://www.un.org/sustainabledevelopment/water-and-sanitation/.

[40] Rubin IL. Break the Cycle of environmental degradation: A commentary. Int Public Health J 2018;10(4):379-88.

[41] Lead. In: Etzel RA, Balk SJ, eds. Pediatric environmental health, 4th edition: Itasca IL: American Academy of Pediatrics, 2019:557-84.

[42] Stillo F, MacDonald Gibson J. Racial disparities in access to municipal water supplies in the American south: Impacts on children's health. Int Public Health J 2018;10(3):309-24.

[43] CDC. Health places. Health effects of gentrification. URL: https://www.cdc.gov/healthyplaces/healthtopics/gentrification.htm.

[44] Frumkin H, Frank L, Jackson RJ. Urban sprawl and public health: Designing, planning, and building for healthy communities, 1st edition. Washington, DC: Island Press, 2004.

[45] Brookings. The changing geography of US poverty. URL: https://www.brookings.edu/testimonies/the-changing-geography-of-us-poverty/.

[46] Rhodes-Bratton B, Rundle A, Lovasi GS, Herbstman J. The relationship between childhood obesity and neighborhood food ecology explored through the context of gentrification in New York City. Int Public Health J 2018;10(4):481-96.

[47] Dragan KL, Ellen IG, Glied SA. Gentrification and the health of low-income children in New York City. Health Aff (Millwood) 2019;38(9):1425-32. doi: 10.1377/hlthaff.2018.05422.

[48] National Center for Education Statistics. The condition of education 2019. URL: https://nces.ed.gov/programs/coe/commissioner.asp.

Rudowitz R, Garfield R, Hinton E. 10 things to know about Medicaid: Setting the facts straight. URL: https://www.kff.org/medicaid/issue-brief/10-things-to-know-about-medicaid-setting-the-facts-straight/.

SECTION ONE: A COMMENTARY

In: Child Environmental Health Disparities ISBN: 978-1-53617-823-4
Editors: IL Rubin and J Merrick

Chapter 2

NATURAL DISASTERS AND VULNERABLE POPULATIONS: A COMMENTARY

I Leslie Rubin[1-5,*], MD, Henry Falk[3,6], MD, MPH and Abby D Mutic[3,7], PhD, CNM

[1]Department of Pediatrics, Morehouse School of Medicine, Atlanta, Georgia, [2]Department of Pediatrics, Emory University School of Medicine, Atlanta, Georgia, [3]Southeast Pediatric Environmental Health Specialty Unit, Emory University, Atlanta, Georgia, [4]Break the Cycle of Health Disparities Inc, Atlanta, Georgia, [5]The Rubin Center for Autism and Developmental Pediatrics, Atlanta, Georgia, [6]Department of Environmental Health, Rollins School of Public Health, Emory University, Atlanta, Georgia and [7]Nell Hodgson Woodruff School of Nursing, Emory University, Atlanta, Georgia, United States of America

[*] Corresponding Author's Email: lrubi01@emory.edu.

[*] Correspondence: I Leslie Rubin, MD, Associate Professor, Department of Pediatrics, Morehouse School of Medicine, Adjunct Associate Professor, Department of Pediatrics, Emory University School of Medicine, Co-Director Southeast Pediatric Environmental Health Specialty Unit at Emory University, Founder, Break the Cycle of Health Disparities Inc, Medical Director, The Rubin Center for Autism and Developmental Pediatrics. 750 Hammond Drive, Building 1, Suite 100, Atlanta, GA 30342, United States. Email: lrubi01@emory.edu.

Every year natural disasters kill around 90,000 people and impact close to 160 million people worldwide. Natural disasters include earthquakes, tsunamis, volcanic eruptions, landslides, tornadoes, hurricanes, floods, wildfires, heat waves and droughts. When a disaster strikes, it has an immediate impact on the physical, biological and social environment with the destruction of property and disruption of human lives. Although a disaster is indiscriminate in whom it affects, poor and medically underserved people, minorities, people with chronic medical problems or disabilities, particularly children and the elderly, bear an unequal burden of the impact. During the initial surge, the health care system is immediately overwhelmed with injuries and acute illness needs, resulting in a sudden and dramatic increase in demand for emergency medical services. Following the initial surge, there are long-term consequences of disasters on the population as well as on the natural environment and the built environment, that have economic, social and political implications on health and wellbeing on individuals, their families, communities and societies. We will explore strategies to prepare for and to minimize the impact of the disasters, particularly on vulnerable populations, and advocate to reduce global warming which contributes significantly to the frequency and intensity of natural disasters.

INTRODUCTION

In this commentary we will present an overview of natural disasters and their consequences, and offer examples that serve to illustrate how different countries and different regions, as well as different populations and communities within a country, suffer disproportionately from the disasters. We will offer strategies in responding to disasters as well as disaster preparedness in order to mitigate the effects of the disasters on human populations, particularly the most vulnerable. In this context we will explore strategies to promote resilience for individuals and for systems to deal with the anticipation of disasters and for positive and constructive responses following the event. We will also address the role of climate change in the frequency and intensity of the natural disasters.

DISASTERS

A natural disaster is an act of nature of such magnitude as to create a catastrophic situation in which the day-to-day patterns of life are suddenly disrupted and people are plunged into helplessness and suffering, as a result, there is a need for medical and nursing care, food, clothing, shelter, and protection against unfavorable environmental factors and social conditions. The impact of the disaster takes a toll on the affected population with an increase in death rate, and with acute injuries and health impacts, as well as long-term physical, emotional and financial consequences for the affected individuals, families, communities and society at large. Every year natural disasters kill around 90,000 people and affect close to 160 million people worldwide (1).

Disasters are divided into two categories:

- *Natural disasters:*
  - Geophysical phenomena such as earthquakes, tsunamis, and volcanos,
  - Climatological/Meteorological conditions such as tornadoes, hurricanes, floods, and wildfires, as well as extreme weather events such as blizzards, droughts, and heat waves
- *Technological disasters* occur as a result of structural failures, such as factory explosions, fires, chemical spills, industrial accidents, transportation accidents, and nuclear accidents, as well as acts of terrorism and civil disturbances, with associated humanitarian refugee crises.

In this commentary we will focus on natural disasters although, as will be seen, there are often associated technological elements that complicate and aggravate the impact of the natural disasters. For the geophysical disasters, we will focus on Tsunamis and Earthquakes and for the climatological or meteorological disasters, we will focus mainly on hurricanes.

PREVALENCE AND CONSEQUENCES

In 1988, WHO established the Center for Research on Epidemiology of Disasters (CRED) to maintain an Emergency Events Database (EM-DAT) of disasters, with the objective of informing humanitarian action at national and international levels in order to improve rational decision-making in disaster preparedness, and provide objective data for assessing communities' needs (2).

In order to be recorded as a natural disaster in EM-DAT, an event must meet at least one of the following criteria:

- Ten or more people reported killed
- 100 or more people reported affected
- Declaration of a state of emergency or
- Call for international assistance.

While EM-DAT is the most comprehensive disaster database available worldwide, there may be some underreporting from certain regions such as from Africa. Be that as it may, the database reported that between 1994 and 2013 there were 6,873 disasters, which claimed a total of 1.35 million lives, with an average of 218 million people affected per year, during that 20-year period. Although earthquakes were the deadliest type of disaster accounting for 45% of deaths, flooding affected the highest number of people, accounting for 50% of the total affected (3).

Figure 1 represents the number of disasters per year from 1900-2018 showing the dramatic increase in natural disasters over the past 50 years (3). This increase in rate and intensity of natural disasters is directly linked to climate change and global warming (4).

Furthermore, there are some areas of the world where particular disasters are more common, for example, along geophysical fault lines such as the Ring of Fire, which is responsible for more than 90% of the world's earthquakes (5). The concerns around flooding are particularly in low-lying coastal cities such as occurred in New Orleans with Hurricane Katrina (6). Some areas of the world are so densely populated that a disaster can take its toll on a larger number of people. Other vulnerable populations live in cities and countries considered poor, with limited financial resources and infrastructural services to prepare or manage the disasters. Members of all communities who are particularly vulnerable are children, older people, those with disabilities or chronic medical conditions, as well as minority populations (7).

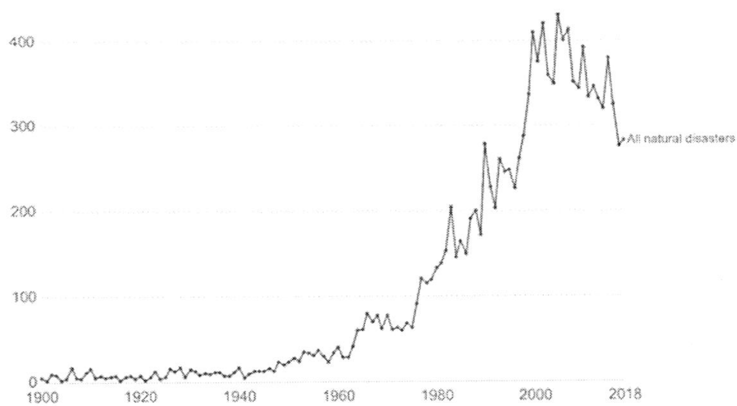

Figure 1. Number of worldwide natural disaster events recorded between 1900 and 2018 (3).

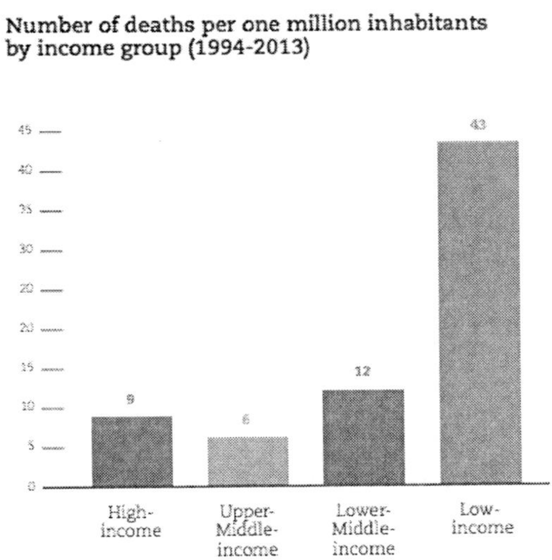

Figure 2. Death rates from disasters in countries with different income levels (8).

Of note is that although the death rates from natural disasters has dropped dramatically because of disaster preparedness strategies, the highest rates of death occur in the poorest populations (3, 8). Figure 2 shows that the death rates for the low-income countries is substantially greater than for the high and middle-income countries. On average, more than three times the number of people died per disaster in low-income countries than in high-income countries, with 332 deaths for the poorest countries versus 105 deaths on average in the richest countries (8).

COST OF NATURAL DISASTERS

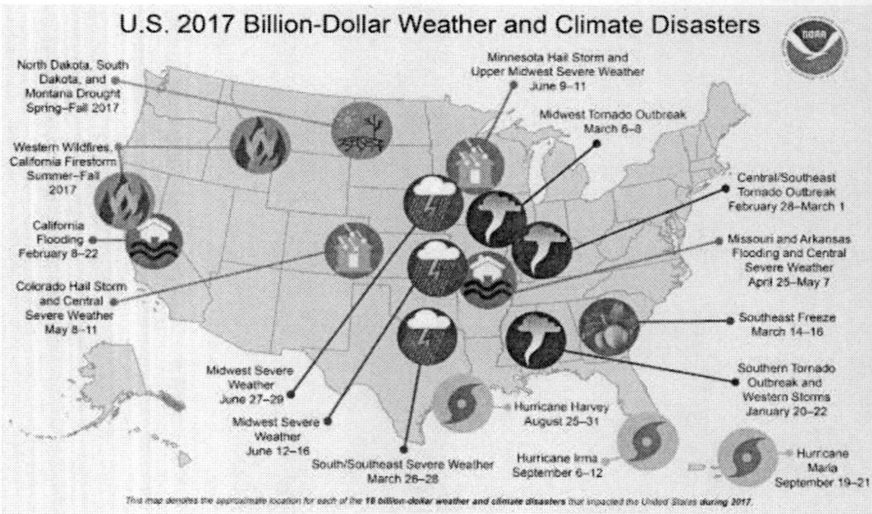

Figure 3. Natural Disasters in the US in 2017 that cost more than $1 billion each (9).

Not only do natural disasters cause much destruction to the natural and built environment with loss of lives and associated physical, emotional and societal disruption, but they come with an economic impact as well. Disasters are very costly – they cause much damage, displace many people and require repairs and restorations to the built environment and community infrastructure, as well as the rebuilding of people's lives and livelihoods. Every year the National Oceanic and Atmospheric Administration of the

USA (NOAA) compiles a list of natural disasters around the world that cost a billion dollars or more (9). The NOAA reports that in 2017, the U.S. experienced a historic year of weather and climate disasters with a total of 16 separate billion-dollar disaster events including: three tropical cyclones, eight severe storms, two inland floods, a crop freeze, drought and wildfire (see Figure 3), with a cumulative cost of over $300 billion (9).

GEOPHYSICAL DISASTERS

Tsunamis (10)

The Indian Ocean tsunami of 2004 was a consequence of an undersea earthquake with a magnitude of 9.1 that struck the coast of the Indonesian island of Sumatra devastating coastal areas as far away as East Africa. Some locations reported that the waves had reached a height of 30 feet or more when they hit the shoreline (11). This tsunami caused massive damage and resulted in more than 225,000 deaths across twelve nations. The lack of food, clean water, and medical treatment, combined with the enormous task faced by relief workers trying to get supplies into some remote areas where roads had been destroyed or where civil war raged, added to the numbers of casualties. Long-term environmental damage was severe, with villages, tourist resorts, farmland, and fishing grounds demolished or inundated with salt water, debris, and bodies. Displacement and damage to infrastructure are important contributors to the human, social, and economic toll of tsunamis. The damage took a long time to repair and cost billions, but psychological scars remain.

The tsunami that hit Japan in 2011 was the consequence of an earthquake with a magnitude of 9.0 located some 80 miles east of the city of Sendai (12). It was not as fatal and the Indian Ocean tsunami of 2004, because of the limited impact and lower population density, with an estimated 28,000 deaths (just over 10% of the toll in the 2004 tsunami). While there was much structural damage to buildings, the greatest concern was the damage to the Fukushima Daiitchi nuclear power plant, which resulted in the release of ionizing radiation into the air, the soil and the water characterizing it as a Technological Disaster as well, with unexpected and cumulative consequences. The severity level of the nuclear emergency at the Fukushima Daiichi facility was estimated to be from 5 to 7 – the highest level on the scale created by the International Atomic Energy Agency – placing the Fukushima accident in the same category as the Chernobyl accident, which had occurred in the Soviet Union in 1986. The repair and recovery of the plant was expected to take about 10 years, but the fallout is expected to last decades. The impacts on humans physically, emotionally and socially are concerning with increase in mortality among vulnerable populations (13).

Earthquakes (14)

The impact on the built environment and on humans from earthquakes is related not only to the intensity, as measured on the Richter Scale, but also has as much to do with the location of the epicenter and its proximity to population centers, as well as the infrastructure of the built environment. We will examine earthquakes in 2 countries in the same year – approximately 1 month apart from each other that serve as a contrast of the consequences in the 2 countries.

Haiti 2010

On January 12, 2010, Haiti was hit by a magnitude of 7.0 earthquake centered about 15 miles southwest of the Haitian capital of Port-au-Prince with a sizable number of aftershocks (15). As a result of the location close to the densely populated capital, as well as vulnerable architectural infrastructure, the devastation was great. Furthermore, being a poor country with limited governmental infrastructure, the country was ill-equipped to deal with such a disaster (16). Buildings collapsed because of lack of building codes, killing or trapping their occupants. Attempts to deal with the disaster by local citizens and organizations, as well as international agencies, including the United Nations, were hampered in their attempts to rescue people who were trapped, and were limited in their ability to provide medical care, food and water because the roads were destroyed or blocked with debris, which further compromised the already limited transportation services. In addition, the failure of the electric power system and loss of communication lines, seriously limited traditional communication services. As a result of this rather chaotic situation, aid was delayed, and more people suffered and died. On a positive note, the country's computer network was functional, and electronic media emerged as a useful mode for coordinating relief efforts and for connecting family members separated by the quake.

An estimated three million people were affected by the quake—nearly one-third of the country's total population, and an estimated 250,000 people died. Over one million people were left homeless in the immediate aftermath and had to live in tent camps with extremely limited resources. Due to major devastation and disruption of civil society, the physical and mental health needs for children were dire (17). Infectious diseases were a major cause of morbidity and mortality in children as well traumatic injuries and malnutrition. Children also suffered abuse and violence with symptoms of posttraumatic stress disorder (PTSD), peri-traumatic stress, depression, anxiety, and food insecurity (18). Of particular concern was the situation of children who had lost their parents and were left vulnerable to abuse and human trafficking. Fortunately, many were adopted by families in other countries, particularly in the United States.

To add insult to injury there was an outbreak of cholera, which was apparently brought to Haiti by members of the UN Peacekeeping Force and, with the cramped and unhygienic living circumstances and lack of adequate healthcare, 283,362 cases of cholera had been reported to the national cholera surveillance system, including 152,816 hospitalizations and 4,856 deaths (19).

The sad reality of this disaster is that it was a massive earthquake that devastated one of the poorest countries in the world and, because of the lack of infrastructure at so many levels, even the best efforts of local and international organizations and agencies were unable to effectively manage the situation. This resulted in a high morbidity and mortality with infrastructural impacts that have residual consequences. At 5 years post-disaster, thousands of people remained displaced and to date, now 10 years later, the people of Haiti are still struggling to recover (20).

Chile 2010

One month after the earthquake in Haiti, on February 27, 2010, there was a magnitude-8.8 earthquake off the coast of south-central Chile, causing widespread damage on land and initiating a tsunami that devastated some coastal areas of the country (21). Although this earthquake was of a much greater magnitude than the one in Haiti, and was associated with a tsunami, the epicenter was about 200 miles southwest of the city and so the impact on the city and its inhabitants was not as devastating. In addition, in stark contrast to the earthquake in Haiti, Chile had experienced previous earthquakes, which prompted the government to institute stringent building codes that significantly limited the damage to buildings. Furthermore, the infrastructure and financial resources of Chile were substantial enough to mobilize more than 10,000 troops to the devastated areas to direct recovery operations and maintain law and order. The Chilean government officials estimated that two million people had been directly affected by the quake and that the earthquake and tsunami resulted in about 500 deaths, in contrast to the number of people affected and the deaths in Haiti (22).

Although the situation was far from perfect and the Chilean Government requested aid from the UN and the US, recovery efforts resulted in a relatively effective return close to previous functioning status by about the middle of 2014. Furthermore, precautions taken in the wake of the 2010 catastrophe were credited with saving lives during a magnitude-8.2 quake and tsunami that occurred in the northern part of Chile in April 2014 and in the September 2015 earthquake off the coast of Illapel. Not only did the people of Chile focus on the practical approach to disasters, they also examined the psychological impact and approaches to ameliorating associated emotional stresses (23).

METEOROLOGICAL DISASTERS

Tornadoes

Tornadoes are violently rotating columns of air extending from the base of a thunderstorm down to the ground and are capable of completely destroying well-made structures, uprooting trees, and hurling objects through the air like deadly missiles. They can occur anywhere, at any time of the day or year but most commonly in the Central Plains and the southeastern US. If there is warning of a tornado, it is advisable to seek shelter with attention focused on the safest place within home (24). However, people living in mobile home are uniquely vulnerable. Although some mobile parks have shelters, this is not common. Because of the short time interval between the warning and the landfall, the effectiveness and functionality of local warning sirens and alert systems are paramount. However, these systems do not always reach everyone at risk, either because of inadequate design or malfunction, leaving residents at risk and vulnerable to the devastation the tornadoes wreak on their fragile homes, leaving them effectively homeless (25).

Heat waves

Heat wave are periods of unusually hot weather that typically last two or more days with temperatures outside the historical averages for a given area. Over the past 5 decades, heat waves, like other natural disasters, have increased in frequency and duration. Typically, the elderly who are socially isolated and living in inner city tenements, which function as 'heat islands' (26), are at greatest risk and those with medical illnesses and taking multiple medications are even more vulnerable. Even brief daily exposure to air conditioning has been found to be effective (27), and public health practice is to establish programs to bring the elderly to air- conditioned malls or other such venues for daily opportunities to cool down (28).

Wildfires

Wildfires are any unplanned fires that burn in forests and other wildlands, such as shrub or grass communities. They can burn millions of acres of land at rapid speeds and can consume everything in their paths, and they are difficult to contain. Concerns about wildfires have increased dramatically with the sharp rise in number and severity of California wildfires (2017-19) and the dramatic events unfolding at this time of writing, in Australia (January 2020) (29). Consequences result in burn injuries from fires, respiratory distress from the acute dramatic rises in particulate air pollutants as a result of the smoke, and the challenges in recovery for communities devastated by the fires. Vulnerable groups accordingly are low income, low resource populations who were forced to move ever further from high cost urban areas and ever closer to at-risk forests; firefighters, emergency responders, and others caught up within ever shifting flames and vulnerable to burn injuries; and individuals with pre-existing cardio-respiratory diseases such as asthma, COPD, and cardiovascular disease who are most heavily impacted by the acute rises in particulate air pollution. The CDC provides valuable information on how to prepare for and protect from wildfires (30). However, given the unpredictable vagaries of huge forest fires, even well-to-do and very prosperous communities, such as those adjacent to Los Angeles, can also find themselves at risk, with sudden changes in wind and temperature superimposed on drought conditions. The consequences from the total annihilation of the built environment from wildfires in the losses for individuals and families are great, as are the impacts on the communities and society, financially and ecologically.

Hurricanes (31)

Hurricanes are considered the most violent storms on Earth and are called by other names, such as typhoons or cyclones, depending on where they occur (Figure 4) (32). The scientific term for all these storms is *tropical cyclone.*

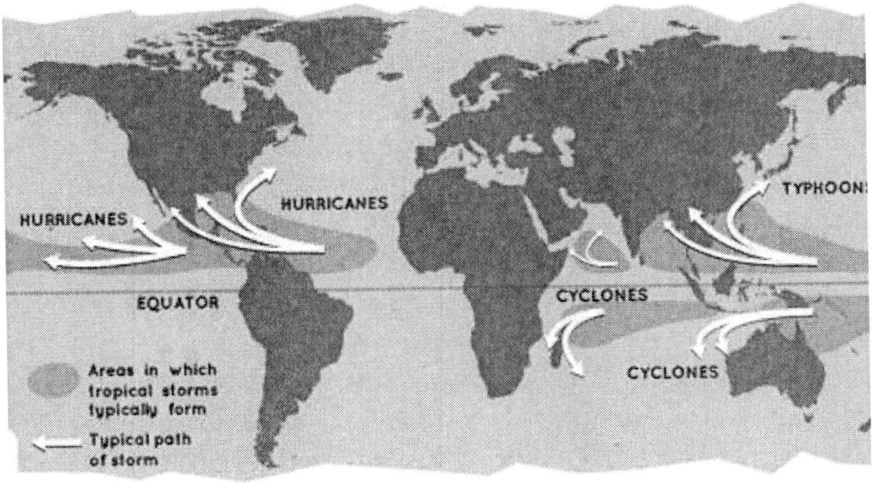

Figure 4. Illustrates the terminology of tropical cyclones depending on where they are located (32).

The classification of hurricanes depends on wind speed, which will determine the consequences on the natural and built environment and on human and animal life (see Table 1) (33).

Table 1. Hurricane categories with associated damage

- *Category 1* – winds 74-95 mph - very dangerous winds will produce some damage – storm surge 4-5 feet
- *Category 2* – winds 96-110 mph - extremely dangerous winds will cause moderate damage– storm surge 6-8 feet
- *Category 3* – winds (major) 111-129 mph - extremely dangerous winds will cause extensive damage – storm surge 9-12 feet
- *Category 4* - winds (major) 130-156 mph - extremely dangerous winds will cause extreme damage – storm surge 13-18 feet
- *Category 5* – winds (major) 157 mph or higher - extremely dangerous winds will cause catastrophic damage – storm surge 19+ feet

According to the Stormfax Weather Almanac 1851-2017 there have been an average of 12 named storms per year with 6.5 per year designated as hurricanes and 2 per year that are classified as major hurricanes of categories 3-5 (34). Of note is that in 2005, the year of Hurricane Katrina, there was a high of 28 storms, with 15 hurricanes and 7 major hurricanes. In 2017 with hurricanes Harvey, Irma and Maria there were 17 storms, 10 hurricanes and 6 major hurricanes (Figure 3).

Individuals living in flood zones and historically impacted coastal areas are obviously most vulnerable. Over the years, the national system of river levees, and the practices of sheltering and evacuation in hurricane affected coastal areas, has provided significant protection in the US, however, these systems have been coming under increasing stress in recent years, thus increasing vulnerability. At the same time, there have been additional increasing risks, which include:

- more frequent high-category hurricanes leading to greater damage and flooding, and overwhelming protective mechanisms (e.g., Hurricanes Katrina, Sandy, Maria, Harvey);
- inadequate insurance and recovery funds, leaving many with long-term vulnerabilities (e.g., Hurricane Maria in Puerto Rico);
- aging levee systems which in some cases are inadequate (e.g., Hurricane Katrina and New Orleans) or whose design is coming under increasing scrutiny because of concerns about effectiveness (e.g., Midwest and Mississippi floods, 2019), leaving increasing numbers of people at risk;
- the increasing impact of climate change.

Hurricane Katrina

With all the storms and hurricanes over the years, Hurricane Katrina stands out as the most devastating and deadliest hurricane since the Galveston hurricane of 1900, which killed an estimated 6,000 to 12,000 people (35). Hurricane Katrina is well recognized as both a natural and technological disaster and demonstrated graphically the triple threat burden: historic health disparities, persistent environmental health risks, and living in a disaster-prone area (36).

Katrina made landfall in southeast Louisiana on August 29, 2005, as a Category 3 hurricane and rapidly became a category 5 hurricane, with sustained winds up to 120 mph making it the third-strongest hurricane ever to affect the United States (37, 38). The resulting storm surge produced waves that were almost three stories high along with 8 to 10 inches of rain that fell along the coast resulting in extensive flooding all along the U.S. Gulf Coast in the states of Mississippi and Louisiana. With much of New Orleans below sea level, the flooding was compounded by more than 50 breaks in levees and floodwalls which resulted in the flooding of 80% of the city. Neighborhoods were destroyed and reduced to scattered rubble. The flooding affected an estimated 77% of the population of Orleans Parish and nearly all the residents of St. Bernard Parish. To further compound matters, at least four Superfund sites in the New Orleans region were hit by the storm and the flooding also resulted in release of noxious chemicals including 575 reports of petroleum or hazardous chemicals spills that were widely distributed by the floodwaters. There were approximately 1,000 deaths from Katrina with 40% from drowning, 25% from injury and trauma and 11% from heart conditions (39).

The destruction of property and displacement of people as well as the disruption and necessary restoration of neighborhoods came at a significant human and financial cost. While the human cost is difficult to determine, the financial cost as estimated by NOAA was at $161 billion – the highest of all hurricanes on record (40).

Although a disaster is indiscriminate, the poor and medically underserved bear an inequitable degree of the burden (41). In Orleans Parish, the mortality rate among black Americans was 1.7 to 4 times higher than whites for all people 18 years old and older (39). These statistics are not surprising in that thousands of low-income minority people of New Orleans, where 69% of the population is African American and 23% live below the poverty line, were living in substandard housing. These areas were totally inundated with the flood waters destroying the fragile buildings and drowning the residents who had not fled the area. Of the other vulnerable groups of people, those who were 75 years old or greater were significantly more likely to be storm victims (37-39).

There had been warnings of the impending storm urging residents of the threatened areas to evacuate to safer areas. The unfortunate reality was that many of the poorer residents of the city, particularly from the most vulnerable areas, did not respond to the warning. Several reasons are postulated. It is possible that some of the residents did not tune into the news or hear the warning because of lack of connection with media. Some may have heard the warning but did not give it credible consideration. Some have previously voiced suspicion and skepticism of the warning sources, displaying general governmental distrust or any source that may appear to be from government (42). Others may not have had reliable sources of transportation or funds necessary to purchase transportation. Some may have been concerned about their potential loss of property or possessions. Finally, some may have been too old, too ill, or physically and mentally unable to take advantage of the opportunity to flee from a potential source of danger. Thus, the people who ultimately lost their lives, their livelihoods, their possessions, their loved ones, their health, their well-being and self-sufficiency were those who were poor, with limited education, limited resources and limited social capital (43).

While more affluent and able citizens heeded the warnings and had sufficient presence of mind and practical resources to leave the threatened areas, thousands of those who remained were herded into the Superdome where they were destined to stay in crowded under-resourced conditions to weather the storm. First-hand reports of the conditions were harrowing with stories of lack of sufficient food, water or medical supplies, lack of sanitation resulting in garbage piling up, and lack of decorum devolving into a dystopian experience (44).

The aftermath for the survivors was dispiriting; with the destruction of homes, loss of possessions and loss of loved ones, they suffered consequences on their physical and mental health with resultant sense of despair and depression affecting children and adults alike. Furthermore, medical resources were limited because hospitals and clinics were also destroyed by the flood, thus taking years to reestablish their lives, their health, their communities, and their sense of well-being.

Another consequence of the widespread damage and destruction was a severe compromise of the public health system in the months after the storm, which, along with substandard living conditions, caused this increased mortality rate, particularly among socially vulnerable groups such as women, children, the elderly, and people with disabilities (38). During the recovery phase there was a 47% increase in the mortality rate from January to June 2006 for the greater New Orleans area. The monthly mortality rate for this time period averaged 91.4 deaths per 100,000 persons, compared with a monthly average of 62.2 deaths per 100,000 for the years 2002–2004 (45).

Children shared many of the environmental and other ubiquitous hazards in New Orleans following the hurricane, such as widespread exposure to mold and heat, vectors, unsafe food, and poor shelter (46). Additionally, there were many concerns that applied specifically to children, such as: the hurried mass transport of very sick neonates and children from New Orleans hospitals during the evacuation of the city; the closing of many pediatric practices in the face of the hurricane, many of which did not reopen; and the disruption of necessary pediatric practices such as newborn screening (47). There were also some unique aspects to the mental health of children caused by the disruption and frenzied evacuation, the fragility of some of the shelters, the separation of thousands of children from their parents and caregivers, the shock of returning to destroyed or heavily damaged homes, and the limited mental health resources for returning or relocated children (48).

Thousands of Gulf Coast families displaced in 2005 by Hurricanes Katrina and Rita were victims of an unprecedented epidemic of chronic medical and mental health problems yet received little appropriate care at the time (49). Even a year later, over half of the New Orleans population had not returned—perhaps as many as three hundred thousand people, many in FEMA-subsidized trailer parks and many in other parts of the country as climate refugees.

While many families who had fled the disaster returned to their original communities, a sizable number stayed in their new locations. They too needed to rebuild their lives and their livelihoods, settle into new school systems and to begin to belong to a community. After Hurricane Katrina, just over one-half of adults returned to the New Orleans metropolitan area, with only one-third returning to their original dwelling. Among the remainder, Texas was the leading location of displaced residents (18%), followed by other locations in Louisiana (12%), other southern states (12%), and elsewhere in the United States (5%). Black adults were considerably more likely to be living elsewhere in Louisiana, in Texas, or other cities in the South (50, 51).

Hurricane Katrina made it evident that natural disasters occur in the same social, historical, and political environment in which disparities in health already exist (36,002042). Furthermore, the racial animosity revealed in a *Washington Post*/Kaiser Family Foundation/Harvard University poll of 680 evacuees, 93% of whom were African American, found that 68% believed the response would have been quicker for White and wealthier people and 61% said that the government does not care about "people like them". These communities experienced social disparities in health before Katrina; their health status was linked to the toxic mix of poverty, poor housing, lack of economic opportunities, and the atmosphere of discrimination in which they lived (52).

The bottom line of the story of Hurricane Katrina and its impact, is that low income, minority people especially the elderly and young children, who live in disaster prone areas of poor neighborhoods, have existing health disparities, or are disproportionately affected by the disaster, are more severely affected by the disaster and have a greater difficulty in recovering from the disaster, if they ever do (36).

Hurricanes in the Caribbean

The vulnerability of the Caribbean islands to natural disasters can be seen in the example of the earthquake in Haiti, referred to earlier in this paper. The islands are small, generally poor and inhabited predominantly by people of African descent. Although some do have agricultural economies, they are heavily reliant on tourism for their main source of revenue. Being in the Caribbean, they are particularly vulnerable to hurricanes. In over 4 consecutive seasons, the Caribbean has experienced several Category 5 Atlantic hurricanes: Matthew (2016), Irma (2017), Maria (2017), Michael (2018) and Dorian (2019). During 2017 alone, 22 of the 29 Caribbean islands were affected by at least one storm, and multiple experienced extreme damage (53). Furthermore, the devastation caused by the hurricanes is not only on the immediate destruction and death toll, but like the example with Katrina or like the earthquake in Haiti, it is long-term. The devastation of the islands' infrastructure with their limited resources, can take years to rebuild. The inevitable stress affects the physical and mental health of the people and, with limited health care resources, can result in an increased morbidity and mortality (54).

These storms and their impact on the Caribbean islands further exacerbate the health and wealth divide, contributing to the cycle of health disparities. The irony of the situation is that the Caribbean islands have an economic base in agriculture and tourism, contributing a miniscule amount of greenhouse gases to the atmosphere, yet, they are in the line of fire from the hurricanes that are coming more frequently and fiercely as a result of the global climate changes that are caused by greenhouse gases from the richer industrialized countries (53). A further example of disparities that play out in the political arena is that of Hurricane Maria that devastated the island of Puerto Rico in 2017. Here, the irony is that in the same year, the Hurricanes that hit the US mainland, Harvey in Texas and Irma in Florida, received substantial federal assistance from the US government through the Federal Emergency Management Agency (FEMA), while Puerto Rico, effectively also part of the USA, did not receive commensurate assistance. This ultimately contributed significantly to the delayed implementation of emergency and rehabilitation services resulting in a further increase in morbidity and mortality (55).

VULNERABLE POPULATIONS

Vulnerable populations can be divided into two major categories: by geographical location, for example on a seismic fault line predisposing to an earthquake, in the equatorial region predisposing to hurricanes and tropical cyclones, or low-lying area predisposing to flooding; or by population characteristics, such as socioeconomic status, age, ethnicity, physical wellbeing, employment, family structure, and housing condition (7, 38 56). Social vulnerability is a measure of both the sensitivity of a population to natural hazards and its ability to respond to and recover from the impacts of hazards. It is a multidimensional construct, not easily captured with a single

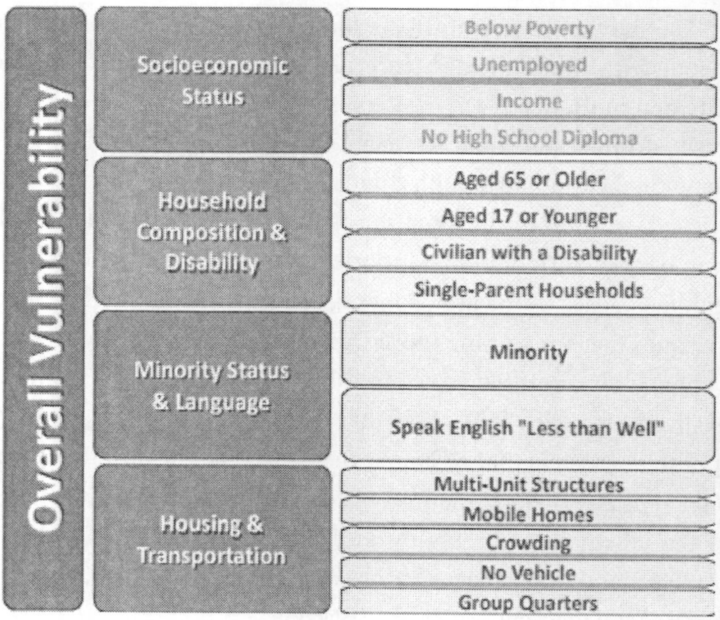

Figure 5. Social Vulnerability Index (7, 38).

variable. There is ample field-based evidence for understanding the characteristics of people and social groups that make them more sensitive to the effects of natural hazards and reduce their ability to adequately respond and recover (57). Social vulnerability also refers to the resilience of communities when confronted by external stresses on human health, such as natural or human-caused disasters, or disease outbreaks. CDC's Social Vulnerability Index uses 15 US census variables at tract level to help local officials identify communities that may need support in preparing for hazards, or recovering from disaster (see Figure 5) (7, 38). The CDC stresses that to mitigate the impact of disasters on at-risk populations, emergency managers must be aware of the social vulnerabilities within their community (58).

DISASTER MANAGEMENT

As seen in the examples of natural disasters presented above, it becomes clear that acute and dramatic devastation to the built environment, the physical environment and the people who are affected, requires an immediate and dramatic response commensurate with the degree and nature of its impact. Furthermore, we need to be cognizant of the vulnerable populations and the long-term consequences. Then follows the steps in rebuilding and restoring a semblance of normality which takes much time. This is particularly the case for vulnerable communities who have limited resources to rebuild or return to their pre-disaster lifestyle. They require a significant level of assistance in recovering their physical and economic security as well as their emotional and social level of wellbeing. This calls for "a holistic community-driven and participatory approach beyond individual survival assistance." (36)

While the damage cannot be undone, there are opportunities to rebuild the affected areas in creative ways that result in safer, healthier, and more resilient communities to better withstand future dramatic events (59). The outcome of this process was described above in the situation of case of the earthquake in Chile, where the potential damage of the earthquake was mitigated by the building codes that had been instituted following previous earthquakes (21, 22). Also, reflected in the reduced death toll from hurricanes (3).

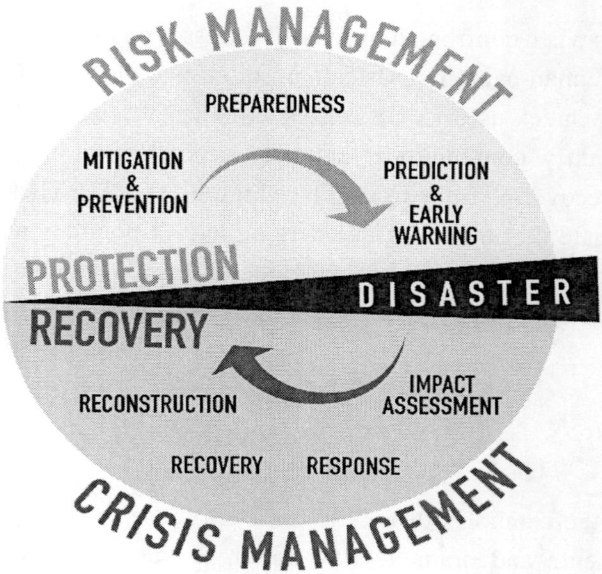

Figure 6. Disaster management cycle (adapted from 60).

Figure 6 represents the elements of the Disaster Management Cycle demonstrating that the way in which we respond to disasters relies upon the crisis management, which informs risk management and disaster preparedness towards mitigation of the impact (60).

Storm Disaster Preparedness

In their paper on the impact of hurricanes in the Caribbean, Schultz et al. make the following recommendations (61):

1. *Communities need to prepare strategically* for the onslaught of stronger storms by revising building codes and redesigning neighborhoods to redress existing socioeconomic inequities in affordable, safe housing and putting in place systems to deal with power outages.

2. *Health care systems need to have emergency response strategies in place* in order to maintain access to lifesaving services and of life-sustaining treatments. This applies to trained personnel as well as hospital facilities.
3. *Enhanced warning systems,* and establishment of available and accessible resources for all citizens with special consideration to vulnerable populations.
4. *Active citizen participation in disaster preparedness and response* can make a big difference in saving lives but also in sharing the burden and working together fosters community cohesion and resilience.
5. *Collaborative conversations and planning process among various segments of society*, including but not limited to health professionals, climate scientists, population health scientists, government agencies and private organizations to advocate for policies that mitigate climate change and develop policies and practices that diminish population health risks and save lives.
6. *Elevate community resilience as an essential public health service* and consequently integrate community resilience measures as performance benchmarks of federal, state, and local health agencies.

Resilience

Resilience is a major factor in surviving a disaster as well as coping with the experiences emotionally, socially and economically in the intermediate aftermath and long-term.

The Composite of Post-Event Well-being (COPEWELL) is a module aiming to support community self-assessments to evaluate factors that influence resilience and incentivize the adoption of interventions that ultimately support National efforts of disaster preparedness, emergency response, and disaster recovery (62). It insists that effective communication must exist in order for communities to function with resilience when faced with a disastrous event (63). Because health care providers are inevitably at the frontlines of health management and patient communication during and after the disasters, the CDC has developed a public health training program entitled, "Crisis & Emergency Risk Communication" (CERC) (64). This multidisciplinary curriculum offers in-person and online instruction for effective disaster communication before, during, and after events. It also offers guidance on handling sensitive topics with special populations and information specific to the type of disaster. It also focuses on the situation of children, who are particularly vulnerable to environmental health risks from disasters and require special attention to effectively address the physical, environmental and biological damage that disasters bring, as well as the emotional trauma that persists long after visible scars have faded.

CONCLUSION

The increasing frequency and severity of natural disasters in the last few decades that is most certainly related to global warming associated with climate change, if unchecked, will undoubtedly continue and become our new reality (4, 65). The lessons learned over the past 20 years since the technological disaster that was the destruction of the World Trade Centers, and the natural disaster that was hurricane Katrina, have resulted in an ever-increasing set of strategies to anticipate and manage natural and technological disasters as they occur and reduce their impact on the environment and on human populations. Yet, the grave concern is that the frequency and severity of the natural disasters will continue to increase towards catastrophic proportions as we have witnessed in the recent fire in Australia (29). Again, although a disaster is indiscriminate in whom it affects, the poor and medically underserved bear an inequitable burden (36, 39, 41, 43, 58). The disastrous storms we have experienced, have not only demonstrated their capacity for destruction of property and impact on human lives, but they come at great cost and have also resulted in an aggravation of injustice with lasting consequences to human health and health disparities.

Our charge, therefore, requires efforts at many different levels involving many difference segments of our global society. We need to confront the imminent threat of global warming (4, 66) we need to continue to focus on the UN Sustainable Development Goals 2030 as a blueprint for action to improve the health of our world (67), all the while preparing for the next disaster wherever it may be and whatever its character (64). Political leaders, health officials, preparedness and response professionals, and community organizations need to act now to develop a shared vision of optimal health for their community. A long-term plan for health and resilience should be a forethought, rather than an afterthought, when a disaster occurs (68, 69).

Acknowledgments

This publication was supported by the cooperative agreement award number 5 NU61TS000237-05 from the Agency for Toxic Substances and Disease Registry (ATSDR). Its contents are the responsibility of the authors and do not necessarily represent the official views of the Agency for Toxic Substances and Disease Registry (ATSDR). The US Environmental Protection Agency (EPA) supports the PEHSU by providing partial funding to ATSDR under Inter-Agency Agreement number DW-75-95877701. Neither EPA nor ATSDR endorse the purchase of any commercial products or services mentioned in PEHSU publications.

References

[1] WHO. Environmental health emergencies. URL: https://www.who.int/environmental_health_emergencies/natural_events/en/.

[2] Center for Research on the Epidemiology of Disasters (CRED). URL: https://www.cred.be/.

[3] Ritchie H, Roser M. Natural disasters. URL: https://ourworldindata.org/natural-disasters.

[4] Union of Concerned Scientists. The science connecting extreme weather to climate change. URL: https://www.ucsusa.org/resources/science-connecting-extreme-weather-climate-change.

[5] USGS. US Department of the Interior. URL: https://www.usgs.gov/media/images/ring-fire.

[6] The World Bank. Which coastal cities are at highest risk of damaging floods? New study crunches the numbers. URL: https://www.worldbank.org/en/news/feature/2013/08/19/coastal-cities-at-highest-risk-floods.

[7] CDC. Social Vulnerability Index (SVI). URL: https://svi.cdc.gov/.

[8] Center for Research on the Epidemiology of Disasters. The human cost of natural disasters. A global perspective. Brussels: CRED, 2015.

[9] NOAA. National Centers for Environmental Information. Billion-dollar weather and climate disasters: Overview. URL: https://www.ncdc.noaa.gov/billions/.

[10] Doocy S, Daniels A, Dick A, Kirsch TD. The human impact of tsunamis: A historical review of events 1900-2009 and systematic literature review PLoS Curr Disasters 2013 April 16. doi: 10.1371/currents.dis.40f3c5cf61110a0fef2f9a25908cd795.

[11] Indian Ocean tsunami of 2004. Encyclopaedia Britannica. URL: https://www.britannica.com/event/Indian-Ocean-tsunami-of-2004.

[12] Rafferty JP, Pletcher K. Japan earthquake and tsunami of 2011. Encyclopaedia Britannica. URL: https://www.britannica.com/event/Japan-earthquake-and-tsunami-of-2011.

[13] Sawano T, Nishikawa Y, Ozaki A, Leppold C, Takiguchi M, Shimada Y, et al. Premature death associated with long-term evacuation among a vulnerable population after the Fukushima nuclear disaster: A case report. Medicine (Baltimore) 2019;98(27):e16162. doi: 10.1097/MD.0000000000016162.

[14] Bolt BA. Earthquake geology. Encyclopedia Britannica. URL: https://www.britannica.com/science/earthquake-geology.

[15] DesRoches R, Comerio M, Eberhard M, Mooney W, Rix GJ. Overview of the 2010 Haiti Earthquake. Earthquake Spectra 2011;27(1):S1–21.

[16] Kligerman M, Barry M, Walmer D, Bendavid E. International aid and natural disasters: A Pre- and post-earthquake longitudinal study of the healthcare infrastructure in Leogane, Haiti. Am J Trop Med Hyg 2015;92(2):448–53. doi: 10.4269/ajtmh.14-0379.

[17] Gupta J, Agrawal A. Chronic aftershocks of an earthquake on the well-being of children in Haiti: Violence, psychosocial health and slavery. CMAJ 2010;182:1997-9.

[18] Dube A, Moffatt M, Davison C, Bartels S. Health outcomes for children in Haiti since the 2010 earthquake: A systematic review. Prehosp Disaster Med 2018;33(1):77-88. doi: 10.1017/S1049023X17007105.

[19] Luquero FJ, Rondy M, Boncy J, Munger A, Mekaoui H, Rymshaw E, et al. Mortality rates during cholera epidemic, Haiti, 2010–2011. Emerg Infect Dis 2016;22(3):410-6. https://dx.doi.org/10.3201/eid2203.141970.

[20] NPR. A 'lost decade': Haiti still struggles to recover 10 years after massive earthquake. URL: https://www.npr.org/2020/01/12/794298546/a-lost-decade-haiti-still-struggles-to-recover-10-years-after-massive-earthquake.

[21] Learning from earthquakes. The Mw 8.8 Chile earthquake of February 27, 2010. EERI Special Earthquake Report, June 2010. URL: https://www.eeri.org/site/images/eeri_newsletter/2010_pdf/Chile10_insert.pdf.

[22] American Red Cross Multi-Disciplinary Team, 2011, Report on the 2010 Chilean earthquake and tsunami response: US Geological Survey Open-File Report 2011-1053. URL: http://pubs.usgs.gov/of/2011/1053/.

[23] Puente S, Marín H, Álvarez PP, Flores PM, Grassau D. Mental health and media links based on five essential elements to promote psychosocial support for victims: The case of the earthquake in Chile in 2010. Disasters 2019l;43(3):555-74. doi: 10.1111/disa.12377.

[24] Eidson M, Lybarger JA, Parsons JE, MacCormack JN, Freeman JI.Risk factors for tornado injuries. Int J Epidemiol 1990;19:1051-6.

[25] Liu S, Quenemoen LE, Malilay J, Noji E, Sinks T, Mendlein J. Assessment of a severe-weather warning system and disaster preparedness, Calhoun County Alabama, 1994. Am J Public Health 1996;86:87-9.

[26] CDC. Heat Islands. URL: https://www.epa.gov/heat-islands.

[27] Kilbourne EM, Choi K, Jones TS, Thacker SB. Risk factors for heat stroke. A case-control study. JAMA 1982;247:3332-6.

[28] Semenza JC, Rubin CH, Falter KH, Selanikio JD, Flanders WD, Howe HL, et al. Heat-related deaths during the July 1995 heat wave in Chicago. N Engl J Med 1996;335:84-90.

[29] Earth Observatory. NASA. URL: https://earthobservatory.nasa.gov/images/event/145600/wildfires-in-australia.

[30] CDC. Wildfires. URL: https://www.cdc.gov/disasters/wildfires/index.html.

[31] Hurricanes. National Oceanic and Atmospheric Administration (NOAA). URL: https://www.noaa.gov/education/resource-collections/weather-atmosphere-education-resources/hurricanes.

[32] Space Place. NASA Science. URL: https://spaceplace.nasa.gov/hurricanes/en/.

[33] Saffir-Simpson Hurricane Wind Scale. URL: https://www.nhc.noaa.gov/aboutsshws.php.

[34] Stormfax Weather Almanac. Atlanat Hurricane Numbers by Year: 1851-2017. URL: http://www.stormfax.com/huryear.htm.

[35] Larson E. Isaac's storm: A man, a time, and the deadliest hurricane in history. New York: Random House, 2000.

[36] Lichtveld M. Disasters through the lens of disparities: Elevate community resilience as an essential public health service. Am J Public Health 2018;108(1):28-30. doi: 10.2105/AJPH.2017.304193.

[37] Kates RW, Colten CE, Laska S, Leatherman SP. Reconstruction of New Orleans after Hurricane Katrina: A research perspective. PNAS 2006;103(40):14653-60. https://doi.org/10.1073/pnas.0605726103.

[38] Flanagan BE, Gregory EW, Hallisey EJ, Heitgerd JL, Lewis B. A social vulnerability index for disaster management. J Homel Secur Emerg Manag 2011;8(1):3. doi: 10.2202/1547-7355.1792.

[39] Brunkard J, Namulanda G, Ratard R. Hurricane Katrina deaths, Louisiana, 2005. Disaster Med Public Health Prep 2008;2(4):215–23.

[40] Hurricane Costs. Office for Coastal Management. NOAA. URL: https://coast.noaa.gov/states/fast-facts/hurricane-costs.html.

[41] Davis JR, Wilson S, Brock-Martin A, Glover S, Svendsen ER. The impact of disasters on populations with health and health care disparities. Disaster Med Public Health Prep 2010;4(1):30–8.

[42] Quinn SC. Hurricane Katrina: A social and public health disaster. Am J Public Health 2006;96(2):204. doi: 10.2105/AJPH.2005.080119.

[43] Zoraster RM. Vulnerable populations: Hurricane Katrina as a case study. Prehosp Disaster Med 2010;25(1):74–8.

[44] Treaster JB. Hurricane Katrina: The Superdome. Superdome: Haven quickly becomes an ordeal. New York Times 2005 Sep 1.

[45] Stephens KU Sr, Grew D, Chin K, Kadetz P, Greenough PG, Burkle FM Jr, et al. Excess mortality in the aftermath of Hurricane Katrina: a preliminary report. Disaster Med Public Health Prep. 2007 Jul;1(1):15-20. doi: 10.1097/DMP.0b013e3180691856.

[46] Falk H, Baldwin G. Environmental health and hurricane Katrina. Environ Health Perspect 2006;114:A12-3.

[47] Barkenmeyer BM. Practicing neonatology in a blackout: The University Hospital NICU in the midst of Hurricane Katrina: Caring for children without power or water. Pediatrics 2006;117:S369-74.

[48] Drury SS, Scheeringa MS, Zeanah CH. The traumatic impact of Hurricane Katrina on children in New Orleans. Child Adolesc Psychiatr Clin North Am 2008;17:685-702.

[49] Burton A. Health disparities: Crisis not over for Hurricane victims. Environ Health Perspect 2006;114(8):A462. doi: 10.1289/ehp.114-a462.

[50] Sastry N, Gregory J. The location of displaced New Orleans residents in the year after Hurricane Katrina. Demography 2014;51(3):753–75. doi:10.1007/s13524-014-0284-y.

[51] Fussell E. The long term recovery of New Orleans' population after Hurricane Katrina. Am Behav Sci 2015;59(10):1231–45.

[52] Survey of Hurricane Katrina evacuees. The Washington Post/Kaiser Family Foundation/Harvard University. URL: https://www.kff.org/wp-content/uploads/2013/01/7401.pdf.

[53] Shultz J, Kossin J, Shepherd J, Ransdell J, Walshe R, Kelman I, et al. Risks, health consequences, and response challenges for small-island-based populations:

Observations from the 2017 Atlantic Hurricane season. Disaster Medicine Public Health Prep 2019;13(1):5-17. doi:10.1017/dmp.2018.28.

[54] Rodríguez-Díaz CE. Maria in Puerto Rico: Natural disaster in a colonial archipelago. Am J Public Health 2018;108(1):30–2. doi: 10.2105/AJPH. 2017.304198.

[55] Kishore N, Marqués D, Mahmud A, Kiang MV, Rodrigues I, Fuller A, et al. Mortality in Puerto Rico after Hurricane Maria. N Engl J Med 2018;379(2):162-70. doi: 10.1056/NEJMsa1803972.

[56] Cutter SL, Boruff BJ. Social vulnerability to environmental hazards. Soc Sci Quart 2003;84(2):242-61.

[57] Cutter SL, Finch C. Temporal and spatial changes in social vulnerability to natural hazards. Proc Natl Acad Sci USA 2008;105(7):2301-6. doi: 10.1073/pnas. 0710375105.

[58] Wolkin A, Patterson JR, Harris S, Soler E, Burrer S, McGeehin M, et al. Reducing public health risk during disasters: Identifying social vulnerabilities. J Homel Secur Emerg Manag 2015;12(4):809-33.

[59] Dzau VJ, Lurie N, Tuckson RV. After Harvey, Irma, and Maria, an opportunity for better health—Rebuilding our communities as we want them. Am J Public Health 2018; 108(1):32–3.

[60] Disaster Management Cycle. Disaster management, emergency response and search and rescue academy. URL: https://sites.google.com/site/dimersarred/disaster-management-cycle.

[61] Shultz JM, Sands DE, Kossin JP, Galea S. Double environmental injustice — climate change, Hurricane Dorian, and the Bahamas. N Engl J Med 2020;382:1-3. doi: 10.1056/NEJMp1912965Comment.

[62] Links JM, Schwartz B, Lin S, Kanarek N, Mitrani-Reiser J, Sell T, et al. COPEWELL: A conceptual framework and system dynamics model for predicting community functioning and resilience after disasters. Disaster Med Public Health Prep 2017;12:127–37.

[63] Schoch-Spana M, Gill K, Hosangadi D, Slemp C, Burhans R, Zeis J, et al. The COPEWELL Rubric: A self-assessment toolkit to strengthen community resilience to disasters. Int J Environ Res Public Health 2019;16(13):2372. doi:10.3390/ijerph16132372.

[64] Centers for Disease Control and Prevention. Emergency preparedness and response. URL: https://emergency.cdc.gov/cerc/index.asp.

[65] Morabia A, Benjamin GC. Preparing and rebuilding after natural disasters: A new public health normal! Am J Public Health 2018;108(1):9–10.

[66] Philipsborn RP, Chan K. Climate change and global child health. Pediatrics 2018;141(6):e20173774.

[67] UN Sustainable Development Goals 2030. URL: https://sustainabledevelopment. un.org/?menu=1300.

[68] Institute of Medicine. Healthy, resilient, and sustainable communities after disasters: Strategies, opportunities, and planning for recovery. Washington, DC: National Academies Press, 2015. URL: https://doi.org/10.17226/18996.
[69] FEMA. National disaster recovery framework. URL: https://www.fema.gov/national-disaster-recovery-framework.

SECTION TWO: BREAK THE CYCLE PROJECTS

In: Child Environmental Health Disparities ISBN: 978-1-53617-823-4
Editors: IL Rubin and J Merrick

Chapter 3

BARRIERS AND OPPORTUNITIES FOR YOUNG CAREGIVERS TO PROVIDE NURTURING CARE IN LOW-INCOME COMMUNITIES OF PARAGUAY

Jimena Vallejos[1,*], MPA, Cassie Landers[2], EdD, MPH and Renata Schiavo[3], PhD, MA, CCL

[1]Columbia University School of International and Public Affair, New York, United States of America

[2]Heilbrunn Department of Population and Family Health, Columbia University Mailman School of Public Health, New York, United States of America

[3]Department of Sociomedical Sciences, Columbia University Mailman School of Public Health, New York, United States of America

---

* Correspondence: Jimena Vallejos, MPA in Development Practice, Columbia University, School of International and Public Affairs, New York, United States. Email: jv2622@columbia.edu; jimevallejos@gmail.com.

ABSTRACT

The United Nations International Children's Fund (UNICEF), the World Bank, and World Health Organization (WHO) suggests a new roadmap for government action and for other programmers and service providers to implement policies and services that help parents and caregivers to provide nurturing care for their children. In Paraguay, despite existing Early Childhood Development (ECD) policies and programs, children, particularly those in poverty, continue to lag behind in many developmental indicators. Young children from low-income households are less likely to have adult members interact with them through stimulation activities, to attend early childhood education centers, or to have three or more books in the home. Furthermore, only 30% of babies are exclusively breastfed for six months, and with limited childcare options, often face greater protection risks from harm. This chapter explores the barriers and opportunities that exist for caregivers to provide nurturing care to their children from pregnancy to age three years in low-income families of Paraguay. Based on a literature review, the mapping of existing ECD programs, and seven semi-structured key informant interviews, this paper analyses the current state of nurturing care in Paraguay. It uses the framework to advocate for the integration of interventions thorough a 'whole child' approach that takes into consideration the multidimensional nature of supports a child and his or her family need, and provides specific recommendations to break the cycle of health disparities with a focus on ECD for young children in Paraguay.

INTRODUCTION

The science of early childhood development (ECD) draws from multiple disciplines including behavioral and social sciences, neuroscience, biology, epigenetics, among others. Since the late 1990s, with ECD programs expanding across the globe, these disciplines have shaped a strong understanding of what constitutes healthy childhood development as well as the potential detrimental consequences for children and for society of failing to support the full development potential of every child (1). At the same time, researchers have developed a solid understanding of what programs and support mechanisms best promote positive outcomes for children. We know today that the brain develops more rapidly in the first three years of life than at any other period in a child's life, and that the architecture of the brain is the result of the interaction between our genetic makeup and the environment, especially our personal experiences early in life (1). It is estimated that, during the critical period of the first three years, a child forms more than one million neuronal connections every second (1, 2). During this rapidly growing period, many of the most basic functions that serve as a foundation for later learning and growth are developing. In order to grow, learn and thrive, children need responsive interactions with their main caregivers complemented by positive experiences and environments that help build a strong brain architecture. This translates into better opportunities for learning, improved health, and higher productivity (3). An additional argument for supporting investment in the early years is evidence favoring that returns on investment for childhood development programs are greater in the early years. Allowing children to build a strong foundation from the very beginning is not only more economical in the long term, but it also promotes a preventive approach instead of an intervention approach, understanding that fixing negative outcomes from disorders of development result in more costly interventions (4).

Along with the growing knowledge of ECD science comes the understanding of factors that can disrupt healthy child development and put children at higher developmental risks. Given that children need nurturing relationships for healthy brain development, experiencing adverse environments and poor interactions puts at-risk children at a further disadvantage and reinforces health and developmental disparities. This may prevent children from developing the skills they need to cope with stress and develop resilience. When children grow up in challenging environments and do not have the support they need, toxic stress may develop as a defense mechanism (1). Prolonged exposure to this type of stress can weaken the architecture of the developing brain (5). The consequences of living in extreme poverty often exposes children to higher levels of toxic stress in early childhood and can have cumulative lifetime effects on learning, future earnings, and health (6).

Experiencing poverty early in life hence significantly contributes to health disparities in childhood as well as in the adult population (7). This is because poverty has profound implications on key life circumstances, such as birth weight, infant mortality, language development, chronic illness, environmental exposure, nutrition, and injury (8). These and other circumstances of poverty can also impact brain development given its association with a higher degree of stress connected with the need to obtain essential resources (food, housing, income) (9), and other challenges in the environment, such as exposure to violence (10).

Poverty adds further stress to the already challenging task of parenting, including the lack of access to parenting knowledge about the needs of the child for responsive and adequate caregiving and access to support networks to address these needs (3, 8). The extent of a family's available resources in terms of financial, social and human capital, can influence a child's potential for reaching his or her optimal development (11). In short, poverty can significantly reduce a caregiver's ability to support, protect, and promote young children's development. This study aims to answer the following question: *What are the barriers for young caregivers to provide nurturing care to their children in low-income communities in Paraguay?* It does so by analyzing the country's ECD landscape under a prominent framework to assess and organize action to promote Nurturing Care to inform future practice and opportunities for integration of programs and policies to achieve optimal development of children (12).

Nurturing care

As described above, the evidence for investing in the early years has grown exponentially. However, even though increased investment has followed, this continues to be insufficient and insignificant portion of government expenditure in most Latin American countries (13). In Paraguay, investment in young children ages 0-5 years represent less than 1% of the Gross Domestic Product (GDP), and less than 7% of total social spending. Furthermore, most of this funding corresponds to education expenses for children 3 years old and above (34%) and health (47%) (14).

An added challenge is that investment does not always translate into better development for children, especially when programs aim to operate at scale where maintaining quality becomes more challenging (15, 16). New evidence is showing the importance of quality implementation in ECD, the fundamental role of multi-sectoral collaboration for its effective implementation, and the need for anchoring any efforts towards improving the development of children under the lens of the domains of the *nurturing care* framework (3).

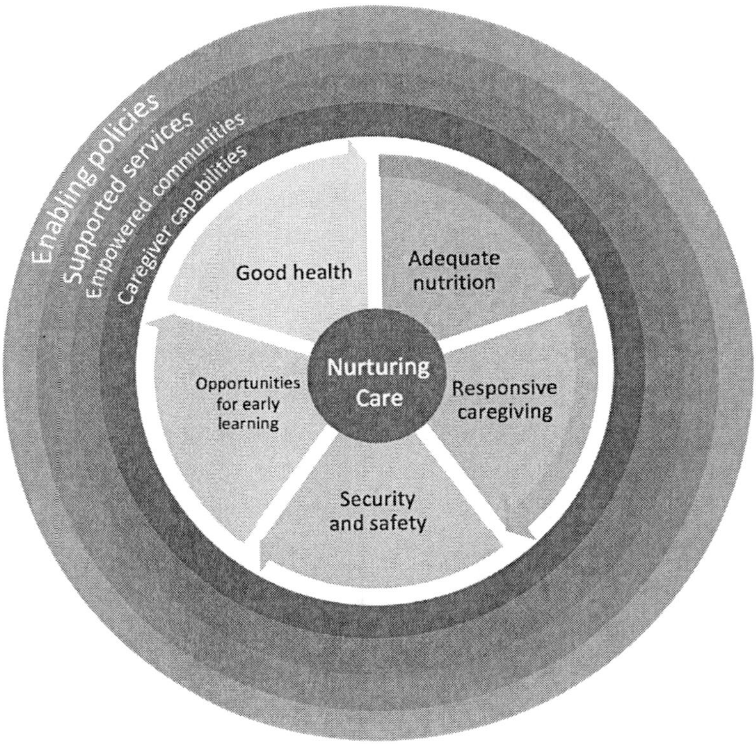

Figure 1. Nurturing care framework. Adapted from (12).

Nurturing care is what children need for healthy development, and it can be understood as "the conditions created by public policies, programs and services ... (that) enable communities and caregivers to ensure children's good health and nutrition and protect them from threats. Nurturing care also means giving young children opportunities for early learning, through interactions that are responsive and emotionally supportive" (12). Even though nurturing care can and must be facilitated and promoted at all levels and contexts (family, school, community, local, and national), it is important to emphasize that "the single most powerful context for nurturing care is the immediate home and care settings of young children often provided by mothers, but also by fathers and other family members, as well as by child-care services" (3).

The Nurturing Care Framework (see Figure 1) developed by United Nations International Children's Fund (UNICEF), the World Bank, and World Health Organization (WHO); provide a roadmap for action which is unique in that it specifically targets the period from pregnancy to the age of three years as the most fundamental period for healthy brain development. The framework calls for a "whole-of-government" and "whole-of-society" approach, outlining principles, strategic actions and guidance for monitoring implementation of progress (12). It is especially relevant for this research considering its age focus, as well as its emphasis on supporting caregivers with the right set of tools and knowledge that allow them to provide nurturing environments to their children. It reinforces the principle that, when provided with adequate and responsive nurturing care, children are more resilient to even the worst effects of adversity (such as extreme poverty). For this reason, guaranteeing nurturing care with healthy and responsive environments is one of the most important actions to help lower a child's stress level as it encourages his or her emotional and cognitive coping mechanisms (12).

The framework in Figure 1 describes the main domains of nurturing care: (a) good health; (b) adequate nutrition; (c) responsive caregiving; (d) security and safety; and (e) opportunities for early learning. It also shows the support system that needs to be in place to ensure that children receive nurturing care starting with caregivers' capabilities, empowered communities who own and defend child development, supportive services that guide caregivers through the challenging task of parenting in this critical period, and moves up to enabling policies that ensure all of the above and guarantee sustainability and continuity of services (12). While the framework articulates the importance of integration across sectors, it also calls for the health sector to play a pivotal role as it is usually the main entry point for care and services during the early years.

In addition to providing guiding principles for policy implementation, the framework for Nurturing Care identifies services and interventions that have proven successful to promote healthy childhood development worldwide under each of the domains presented above (3, 12). While it is evident that different governmental and non-governmental institutions play different roles for the implementation and delivery of such services, this approach uses a whole child perspective allowing for integration of services based on a child's needs for optimal development rather than based on institutional capacities. This study is unique in that it assesses ECD in Paraguay using the Nurturing Care framework to make a case for integration of services at all levels and provide a series of recommendation for improving opportunities for caregivers in poor households to provide nurturing care to their children.

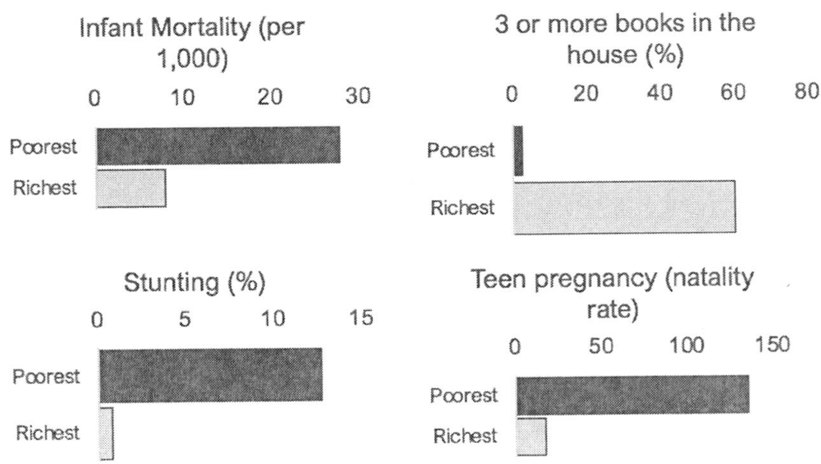

Figure 2. Paraguay ECD indicators by wealth quintiles (17).

Early childhood development in Paraguay

Despite noticeable progress in health, nutrition and education enrollment in Paraguay, children's developmental outcomes vary significantly depending on where children grow up and their socio-economic status (see Figure 2). Children in the poorest areas are at greater risk for experiencing infant mortality or stunting and malnutrition. They are also much less likely to have adult members interact with them through stimulation activities (only 2 in every 10 children in the poorest households receive stimulation), to attend early childhood education centers, or to have three or more books in the house. Furthermore, they are more likely to be born to an adolescent mother and given that low-income families have limited childcare options children are often at greater risks of needing protection (17).

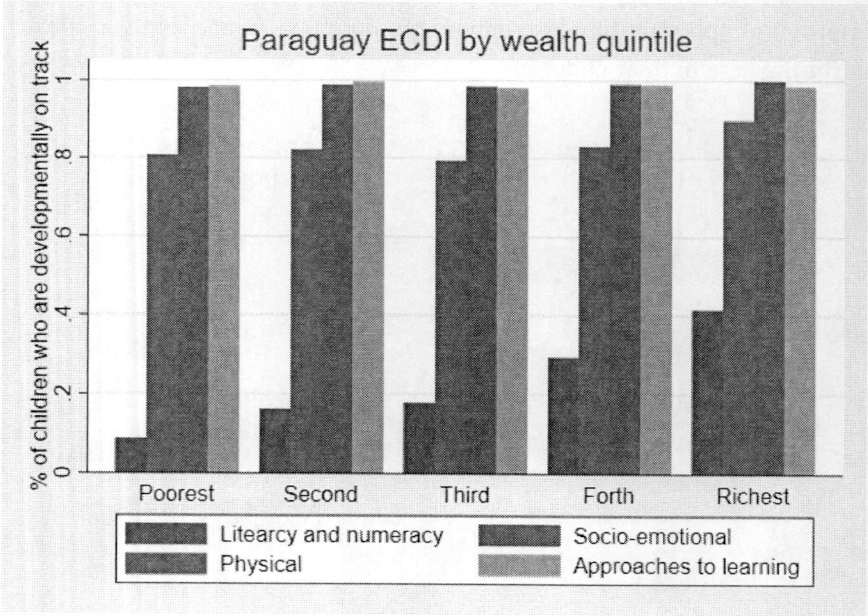

Figure 3. Distribution of ECDI scores in Paraguay by wealth quintiles (17).

Paraguay presents an overall 81.9 score in UNICEF's Early Childhood Development Index (ECDI) (17, 18). Figure 3 shows the distribution of ECDI scores by wealth quintiles in Paraguay. Even though most children are developmentally on track in terms of physical development (97,6%) and approaches to learning (95,8%), the development domains of literacy and numeracy, and socio-emotional development show greater variation and lags in development disproportionally affect children in the lowest wealth quintiles (17).

In recent years, the increased interest in ECD has led to the development of a national plan for early childhood, the *Plan Nacional de Desarrollo Integral de la Primera Infancia* (PNDIPI) in 2011 and the launching of multiple ECD programs by public, private and civil society sectors. The PNDIPI was pivotal for introducing ECD in the national agenda and for complementing a legal and policy framework with clear action towards young children (see annex 1 for Paraguay's legal and programmatic ECD landscape). It set important targets for putting children at the center for intervention and called for a multi-disciplinary and collaborative approach to address young children's needs. One of its most important components was the establishment of a national commission on early childhood, known as the *Comisión Nacional de Primera Infancia* (CONPI) as the key promoter agency for the implementation of the plan. This commission is formed by representatives of the Ministry of Health, the Ministry of Education and Science, and the Ministry of Childhood and Adolescence who rotate leadership positions. However, to date CONPI has played primarily a coordination function. As such, it is not an independent body and lacks the autonomy to demand implementation, influence policy and dictate fundamental aspects of the ECD agenda such as demanding funding allocation and monitoring and evaluation of programs.

The PNDPI will undergo an evaluation process at the end of 2019. Importantly, however, reports from key informant interviews, as well as a limited number of publications available on the subject, express important concerns in the translation of the plan from policy to implementation and sustainability (19).

OUR STUDY

A review of the literature was conducted to develop an understanding of the key concepts addressed in the research. The starting point was the recently published document *Nurturing care for early childhood development: A framework for helping children survive and thrive to transform health and human potential* (11), which serves as the guiding framework for this research. The reference list of this document was reviewed and included to expand the research. In addition, Columbia University Library Database was searched using the terms "brain development," "early childhood development," and "nurturing care" "poverty and children health disparities," "ECD policies in Latin America," "Early Childhood Development in Paraguay" from 2000 through 2019.

Web searches on local websites of UNICEF Paraguay, Ministry of Childhood and Adolescence, Ministry of Education and Science, Ministry of Health as well as non-profit organizations was conducted to obtain program and policy information specific to Paraguay. Furthermore, the dataset from UNICEF's Multiple Indicator Cluster Surveys conducted in 2016 was downloaded from UNICEF's website and used to analyze and report ECD outcome indicators from Paraguay.

Finally, a series of in-person and remote key informant interviews with selected participants working in the ECD sector of Paraguay were conducted. The key informant interviews elicited stakeholder opinions on the relevance, effectiveness, efficiency, sustainability and impact of early childhood development programs in Paraguay, with special emphasis on opportunities and barriers for young caregivers to provide nurturing care. A detailed list of the institutions represented during the interviews as well as the guiding questions are included in annex 2. The names have not been included for confidentiality purposes. Data triangulation was achieved by interviewing a range of stakeholders at different levels from a variety of institutions and reviewing a wide range of documents.

Findings are organized under the main domains of the Nurturing Care framework with the intent of identifying the barriers for young caregivers to provide nurturing environments and highlight opportunities for integration and clear recommendations that can be adopted by policy makers and program implementers (12).

FINDINGS

Barriers for caregivers to provide nurturing care

This section assesses the main barriers to implementation of nurturing care from the perspective of practitioners and policy makers in Paraguay looking at both household and national level barriers. The end objective is to identify clear opportunities for aligning existing efforts and incorporating recommendations based on the Nurturing Care framework. For reference, findings from key informant interviews are highlighted in bold, and dimensions of the framework are marked in italics.

While it is important to understand the specific needs of children in the different domains of nurturing care, the first finding that became evident is how closely interrelated these domains are. This reinforces the idea that the inability of caregivers to fulfill needs within one domain, puts children at a greater risk in other domains as well (20). For example, time and caregiver's availability due to caregivers working 15-18 hours outside of the home was identified as a barrier for *responsive caregiving*. However, having caregivers on such a stressful schedule due to financial need is likely to also affect the caregivers' capacity to provide *security and safety* as children are often left in someone else's care because of the work commitment of the primary caregiver. This may, at the same time, limit the caregivers' ability to seek timely healthcare and appropriate treatment when the child is ill, affecting the caregiver's ability to provide *good health*. What follows is an attempt to organize findings from the interviews under each domain, with the caveat that many of these barriers and challenges affect and relate to each other:

1.1. *Good health*: barriers to good health at the household level include,

- **Large percentage of teen pregnancies** among low-income caregivers put children at greater risk for low-birth weight and, consequently, poor development outcomes (21). Every day two girls between 10 and 14 years old give birth in Paraguay (22). These numbers are alarming given that a pregnancy in early adolescence is most often the result of sexual abuse (22). In addition, the adolescent fertility rate is of 72 births for every 1,000 women ages 15 to 19 years, with adolescent mothers in this age range representing 20% of total births (17). When disaggregated by region, language spoken at the home and years of study, the adolescent fertility rate goes up ranging from 84 to 164 births every 1,000 women ages 15 to 19 years, showing again a large disparity gap for adolescents in the poorest areas (17, 22).
- **Extreme climate events:** Extreme heat waves and periods of flooding are the largest environmental threats in Paraguay (23). While flooding has been a challenge throughout history, the problem has exacerbated in recent years with more frequent floods and a larger number of families affected by these extreme weather events. Vulnerable populations are often displaced and face increased exposure to weather related diseases while experiencing additional sources of stress. Paraguay presents a vulnerability index classified as *extreme* and has been ranked as the 8th most vulnerable country to climate change Latin America and the most vulnerable in South America (24). In 2019, over 49,637 families have been affected by flooding, with at least 11,144 families experiencing displacement (25). In the context of these emergencies, ECD interventions are challenging to implement and national strategies for dealing with climate change, including Paraguay's, rarely include an intervention approach for the early years (26).
- **Lack of hygiene at the household level:** This barrier is reinforced by an overall lack of awareness and limited education in low income families as addressed in *1.3.* below.

1.2. *Nutrition*: barriers to nutrition at the household level include,

- **Limited breastfeeding practices**: only 30% of children are exclusively breastfed until six months (17). Mothers rarely receive sufficient guidance and support regarding the benefits and importance of breastfeeding for the developing child.
- **Malnutrition:** Paraguay achieved significant progress in reducing the rural-urban gap in nutrition since the mid 1990s until 2012 (27). However, stunting levels still remain at 6% in children 0-5 years (17). Today, in line with the global phenomenon, the country is beginning to co-exist with the challenges of eliminating undernutrition while increasingly having to pay attention to the **challenge of childhood obesity** with highly unbalanced diets. This is particularly worrying in vulnerable populations such as indigenous community that migrate to urban areas (28).

1.3. *Responsive caregiving*: barriers to responsive caregiving at the household level include,

- **Time** and caregivers' availability: As mentioned above, low-income caregivers who have to spend a significant portion of their days at work and leave their children under the care of others (often grandmothers or older children) face time constraints for spending quality time with their children.
- Intrusion of **mobile technology** into parental interactions was increasingly recognized as a challenge as parents tend to use technology to keep children entertained (29). The framework recognizes the added premium that strong cognitive and social abilities that are development in the early years will continue to hold in our increasingly digital world. However, interventions must also stress the importance of human interactions with the main caregivers as the most fundamental factor to ensuring strong development in early childhood.
- **Culture:** Two important components were raised under culture. One is a culture of physical punishment which is addressed further in *1.5.*, and another commonly shared concern is the idea of

demonstrating affection as a symbol of vulnerability. Children need love and affection. Boys and girls alike. An important finding at the national level highlights the need for gender sensitivity. Most of the concern was expressed around girls and their vulnerability to sexual abuse (also addressed in *1.5.);* however, this finding also calls attention to possible risks regarding the way that children are socialized into different gender roles at a very early age and its possible negative effects on children's development (30). Culture is also highly linked to opportunities for learning, for example, understanding the role and importance of play. This is addressed in the following point.

1.4. *Opportunities for early learning*: barriers to opportunities to early learning at the household level include,

- **Lack of awareness of the importance of play:** Caregivers often want to play with their children but there is a lack of awareness on the importance of early and responsive interactions, and the role of play in children's development. As it was put in one of the interviews "fathers wait until their child is old enough to play football, at that time, it can be late already." The value play and the implications of spending time playing with children, particularly in ages 0 to 3 years, have for the development of children is not internalized in most caregivers.
- **There is an existing notion that school, and learning, starts in pre-school**. There is a lack of awareness that learning begins at home and not when children enter the education system. In rural areas, children wait to be the same age to go to school together.
- **Location of early childhood education services**: Even if pre-school or early care services for young children are available, 3-year-old children cannot walk a kilometer to school as compared to school-age children.

1.5. *Security and safety:* barriers to safety and security at the household level.

- **Lack of basic income:** extreme poverty was identified as the main barrier to nurturing care in all interviews. Income poverty and extreme poverty affect 24.2% and 4.8% of the population respectively (31). This barrier significantly affects the ability of caregivers to provide nurturing care due to higher levels of stress, reduced levels of education, and lack of access to jobs as explained above.
- **Poor housing conditions and overcrowded households**: Paraguay has a household deficit of 50% with housing lacking both in terms of quantity and quality. The demand quantity is concentrated in urban areas due to large populations living in informal settlements whereas quality housing deficit in need of improvements and expansion is higher in rural areas (32). The housing deficit is further exacerbated by the challenges resulting from flooding and an increase in the number of families and children living in informal and often insecure, urban settlements.
- **Culture of punishment**: over 50% of children 1 to 14 years of age experience physical punishment or psychological aggression (17). Families replicate what they know from their own experiences growing up' thus perpetuating the cycle of punishment.

1.6. *System barriers:* In addition to the barriers corresponding to the different domains within the Nurturing Care Framework, several barriers were identified at a systems and policy level. These relate to the implementation, monitoring and scaling up of national programs and policies. They include:

- The PNDIPI policy, which is in its last year of implementation, was identified as an opportunity and barrier at the same time. The policy has been questioned for its **lack of accountability**. While it was important for introducing new early childhood development programs, creating the CONPI, and suggest articulation across government actors, there is no clear evaluation or accountability mechanisms in place to understand how successful the plan has been in advancing and improving ECD.

- More importantly, there is no evidence that this plan **has translated into an integrated approach to child development**. In spite specific language in the plan advocating for interinstitutional collaboration, programs across ministries and institutions have mostly continued to work and develop in silos. Efforts to integrate operate primarily at a pilot stage. Furthermore, programs are often centralized at the ministerial level, leaving little capacity and discretion for implementation at the local level.
- Another important barrier is **institutional weakness.** This is expressed both in **limited multi-sector coordination and implementation** as well as in the limited transition of learning and progress from one administration to the next. While a right-based approach and a multi-sectorial approach is often discussed, programs in the field show little connection to each other.
- Finally, the Nurturing Care framework highlights the importance of funding that is "sustainable, equitably distributed, efficient and flexible" (11). The last identified barrier to nurturing care is the **sustainability of the current ECD policy**. Financing of ECD occurs primarily through projects, multilateral cooperation, and yearly allocations rather than being embedded as part of the regular national budget.

Parents and other caregivers are the main force and resources for early childhood development in the first three years of life. For this reason, equipping them with the knowledge, capabilities and resources to provide nurturing care for their children in these five domains is essential for ensuring that they reach their full potential. These findings shed light on the need to strengthen awareness raising services and streamlining information for caregivers in low-income families. Raising awareness is an important way of developing accountability mechanisms so that, in turn, government can become more efficient. Caregivers who know that providing nurturing environments for their children is a clear pathway towards breaking the cycle will be more likely to demand and use ECD services (see Figure 4).

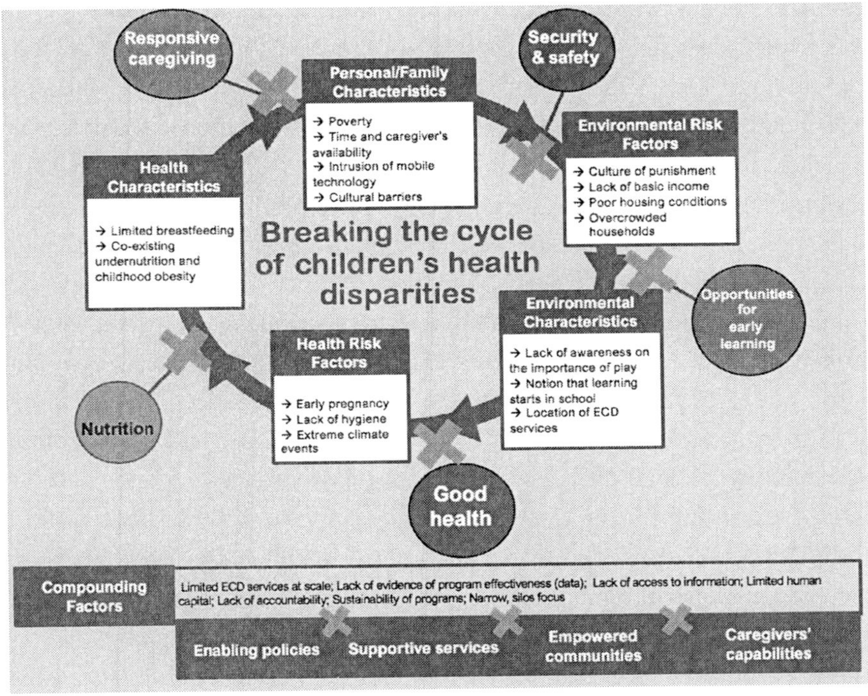

Figure 4. Using the Nurturing Care framework to break the cycle of health disparities (12).

Opportunities for caregivers to provide nurturing care

While there are many barriers at the family, community and policy level to promote nurturing care in Paraguay, the literature review and interviews also revealed many opportunities to strengthen nurturing care at all these levels. Using the Nurturing Care Framework to organize and prioritize actions provides an opportunity in and of itself, but additional opportunities were identified and are important to take advantage of the momentum.

In 2018, the government of Paraguay in partnership with the Interamerican Development Bank and UNICEF launched two important initiatives. First, a new program, *Modelo de Atención Integral del Desarrollo Infantil Temprano (MAIDIT*). The program aims to deliver ECD services through a model based on the public health system. It incorporates important components included as key practices in the Nurturing Care framework such as the arrangement of programs and policies under a continuum of care with universal, targeted, and intensive services based on individual families' needs (12). Second, the government of Paraguay launched the *Sistema Nacional de Protección Social ¡Vamos!* (SPS), a national social protection system as its primary platform for organizing its social policy at the end of 2018. The SPS organizes public action by lifecycle with a strong emphasis on early childhood. Both of these platforms present a unique opportunity for this study. Using Nurturing Care can provide further guidance for implementation of the MAIDIT program as it continues to roll out in 10 regions of Paraguay in the next few years (33) and for the SPS as it is rolled out nationally (34). The PNDIPI and its upcoming evaluation was also highlighted as an opportunity given that it has provided extensive training for the early childhood workforce and put the CONPI in place. While there is much room for improvement, these mechanisms are very adaptable to the Nurturing Care Framework. Finally, it was largely recognized that in the South American region there are examples of best practices related to successful ECD policies that have been widely studied such as national ECD plans of Chile (Chile Crece Contigo), Colombia (De Cero a Siempre) and Uruguay (Uruguay Crece Contigo) that have been successful in improving child development outcomes indicators with a special emphasis on vulnerable populations (See Annex 3). An analysis of best practices of the region and exploring potential partnerships for adaptation and replication provide a unique opportunity for Paraguay to strengthen its current policies and programs.

DISCUSSION

This review presents a comprehensive analysis of the barriers and opportunities for parents and caregivers in Paraguay to provide nurturing care to their children in the first three years of life. It uses key findings from stakeholders' interviews combined with a review of the literature to highlight important gaps in guaranteeing the optimal development of children during this critical period. Below, I present key recommendations that emerged from the research under the five strategic actions recommended for governments in the framework for Nurturing Care (11):

1) *Focus on families and their communities*:
   - The need to increase the knowledge and awareness of caregivers as well as their capabilities through providing timely information and adequate support systems for everyone must continue to be the primary vision for improving and ensuring the development of services for children in the early years, particularly for the most vulnerable populations.
   - Participatory processes for increased community involvement can bring new ideas not only for increasing awareness on nurturing care but for finding new practices and new ways of engaging in the way we care about children.
2) *Lead and invest*: Take into account regional examples of ECD laws and programs that guarantee long term financing and facilitate the integration of services across sectors. The Social Protection System is an important first step, but quality implementation at scale is key.
3) *Strengthen services*: This analysis identifies key barriers at the family, community and system's level. Organizing them under Nurturing Care provides a strong case for the need of improving efforts towards the integration of services as well as the introduction of new tools and mechanisms to facilitate such process. Global experiences show that interinstitutional ECD commissions, such as the CONPI, can play a key part of the coordination for the integration of services. Looking at regional examples can further inform how to improve the implementation capacity of this important unit and support the definition of a strong management model that guarantees access to services through vertical and

horizontal coordination across governmental ministries, particularly for policy efforts such as the SPS.

4) *Monitor progress*: Integration needs to happen not only at the program level, but also in terms of sharing information around quality monitoring. Finding creative ways to make families accountable and increase their demand for services is an important step in improving the effectiveness of programs.
5) *Use data and innovate*: It is important to determine ways in which the data that is collected today at the family level can be used to inform actual needs and promote an ecosystem to nurture innovative solutions from different sectors. Furthermore, the integration of data information systems is an important step in efforts of intersectoral collaboration.

Expanding these lines of actions and taking into account the insights from this study can help overcome the barriers to nurturing care and break the cycle of health and developmental disparities for low-income children in Paraguay as it provides a roadmap for improving the current ECD landscape and transition into a holistic approach with caregivers and children at the center of any intervention (see Figure 4).

CONCLUSION

Placing emphasis on parents and caregivers' capabilities to provide nurturing environments for their children is fundamental for their optimal development. Paraguay has made good progress to establish policies and programs that promote ECD, however, its most vulnerable population continue to lag behind in many indicators of early childhood development. The inability to ensure optimal development of children has negative and long term social and economic implications for the country. For this reason, it is fundamental that current increasing interest in ECD and existing policies be translated into effective and high-quality implementation. The Nurturing Care Framework provides a roadmap to organize public action with a strong emphasis on developing and empowering parents and caregivers' skills and capabilities.

Acknowledgments

A special thank you to Dras Cassie Landers and Renata Schiavo for their guidance, support and encouragement for the research in this topic and in general for encouraging me in the pursuit of a career in this fascinating field. I also recognize the invaluable support and guidance of *Break the Cycle 14* faculty, mentors, and fellows. This work was conducted in honor and memory of Maren Castro Villagrana Jakobsmeier, SIPA MPA '18, a student dedicated to making the world a better place for children.

References

[1] Center on the Developing Child at Harvard University. From best practices to breakthrough Impacts: A science-based approach to building a more promising future for young children and families, 2016. URL: http://www.developingchild.harvard.edu/.

[2] Nelson CA, Zigler EF. The neurobiological bases of early intervention. In: Zigler ED, Shonkoff JP, Meisels SJ, eds. Handbook of early childhood intervention. Cambridge: Cambridge University Press, 2000:204–28.

[3] Britto PR, Lye SJ, Proulx K, Yousafzai AK, Matthews SG, Vaivada T, et al. Nurturing care: promoting early childhood development. Lancet 2017;389(10064):91–102.

[4] Heckman JJ. Skill formation and the economics of investing in disadvantaged children. Science 2006;312(5782):1900–2.

[5] Shonkoff JP, Garner AS, Siegel BS, Committee on Psychosocial Aspects of Child and Family Health; Committee on Early Childhood, Adoption, and Dependent Care; Section on Developmental and Behavioral Pediatrics. The lifelong effects of early childhood adversity and toxic stress. Pediatrics 2012;129:e232–46.

[6] Robinson LR, Bitsko RH, Thompson RA. CDC grand rounds: Addressing health disparities in early childhood. MMWR 2017;66(29):769-72.

[7] Brooks-Gunn J, Duncan JG. The effects of poverty on children. Future Child 1997;2:55–71.

[8] Pediatrics Council on Community (PCC). Poverty and child health in the United States. Pediatrics 2016;137(4):e20160339.

[9] Blair C, Granger DA, Willoughby M. Salivary cortisol mediates effects of poverty and parenting on executive functions in early childhood. Child Dev 2011;82(6):1970–84.

[10] Evans GW. The environment of childhood poverty. Am Psychol 2004;59(2):77-92.

[11] Urke HB, Contreras M, Matanda DJ. The influence of maternal and household resources, and parental psychosocial child stimulation on early childhood development: A cross-sectional study of children 36-59 months in Honduras. Int J Environ Res Public Health 2018;15(5:926.

[12] World Bank, UNICEF, WHO. Nurturing care for early childhood development: A framework for helping children survive and thrive to transform health and human potential 2018. URL: http://apps.who.int/iris/bitstream/handle/10665/272603/9789241514064-eng.pdf.

[13] López N, Cursio J, Frenkel J, Aprile M, Cetrángolo F, Goldschmit A, Robba M, Sotelo JM. La inversión en la primera infancia en América Latina: Propuesta metodológica y análisis en países seleccionados de la región. United Nations International Children's Emergency Fund (UNICEF), 2015. URL: http://www.sipi.siteal.iipe.unesco.org/sites/default/files/sipi_publicacion/sipi_ispi_boletin.pdf [Spanish].

[14] López N, Cursio J, Frenkel J, Aprile M, Cetrángolo F, Goldschmit A, Robba M, Sotelo JM. La inversión en la primera infancia en América Latina: Propuesta metodológica y análisis en países seleccionados de la región – Ficha Paraguay. United Nations International Children's Emergency Fund (UNICEF), 2015. URL: http://www.sipi.siteal.iipe.unesco.org/sites/default/files/sipi_publicacion/sipi_ispi_paraguay_v2.pdf [Spanish].

[15] Yousafzai AK, Aboud FE, Nores M, Kaur R. Reporting guidelines for implementation research on nurturing care interventions designed to promote early childhood development. Anna NY Acad Sci 2018;1419(1):26–37.

[16] Britto PR, Singh M, Dua T Kaur R, Yousafzai AK. What implementation evidence matters: Scaling-up nurturing interventions that promote early childhood development. Anna NY Acad Sci 2018;1419(1):5–16.

[17] UNICEF. Encuesta de indicadores múltiples conglomerados MICS Paraguay 2016. URL: https://bit.ly/2E2qJac [Spanish].

[18] Loizillon A, Petrowski N, Britto P, Cappa C. Development of the Early Childhood Development Index in the MICS Surveys. New York: Data and Analytics Section, Division of Data, Research and Policy UNICEF, 2017. URL: http://mics.unicef.org/files?job=W1siZiIsIjIwMTcvMDkvMTUvMjEvMTUvNDMvMzc4L01JQ1NfTWV0aG9kb2xvZ2ljYWxfUGFwZXJfNi5wZGYiXV0&sha=85c096f0b2c5b0c8.

[19] Sosa Walder P. Early childhood education policy in Paraguay: Identifying the main obstacles of the implementation of the National Plan for the Integral Development of Early Childhood 2011-2020 from a policymaker's perspective. London: University College of London (UCL), Institute of Education, 2018. [Spanish].

[20] Sameroff A. A unified theory of development: a dialectic integration of nature and nurture. Child Dev 2010;81(1):6–22.

[21] The Schuyler Center for Analysis and Advocacy. Teenage births: Outcomes for young parents and their children, 2008. URL: https://www.scaany.org/documents/teen_pregnancy_dec08.pdf.

[22] Dobrée P, Escobar R, Soto C, Soto L. Embarazo y maternidad de niñas en Paraguay Asunción: Centro de Documentación y Estudios (CDE), 2018. URL: http://www.cde.org.py/wp-content/uploads/2018/12/Embarazo-niñas-FINAL-web-1.pdf [Spanish].

[23] PNUD Paraguay. Cambio Climático: Riesgos, vulnerabilidad y desafío de adaptación en el Paraguay, 2017. URL: http://www.py.undp.org/content/paraguay/es/home/library/crisis_prevention_and_recovery/cambio-climatico--riesgos--vulnerabilidad-y-desafio-de-adaptacio.html [Spanish].

[24] Cooperación Andina de Fomento (CAF). Vulnerability Index to climate change in the Latin American and Caribbean Region, 2014. URL: scioteca.caf.com/bitstream/handle/.../509/caf-vulnerability-index-climate-change.pdf.

[25] Dirección de Información Epidemiológica Dirección General de Vigilancia de la Salud DGVS-MSPBS. Reporte de inundaciones: Vigilancia intensificada en inundaciones, 2019. URL: http://www.vigisalud.gov.py/files/boletines_inundaciones/SE24_7_2019_Boletin_Inundaciones.pdf [Spanish].

[26] Secretaría del Ambiente, Oficina Nacional de Cambio Climático. Estrategia Nacional de Adaptación al Cambio Climático. Asunción, Paraguay: Secretaría del Ambiente, 2015:43. [Spanish].

[27] Ervin PA, Bubak V. Closing the rural-urban gap in child malnutrition: Evidence from Paraguay, 1997–2012. Econ Hum Biol 2019;32:1–10.

[28] Arza Insfrán EA, Collante Lavand V, Sanabria M, Acosta J, Morínigo Martínez M, Arza Insfrán EA, et al. Double burden of malnutrition in mothers and children under five years of age in two indigenous communities of the Central Departament. Anales de la Facultad de Ciencias Médicas (Asunción). 2018;51(3):53–60.

[29] Kildare CA, Middlemiss W. Impact of parents' mobile device use on parent-child interaction: A literature review. Comput Hum Behav 2017;75:579–93.

[30] Lytton H, Romney DM. Parents' differential socialization of boys and girls: A meta-analysis. Psychol Bull 1991;9(2):267.

[31] Dirección General de Estadística, Encuestas y Censos (DGEEC). Principales resultados de pobreza monetaria y distribución de ingresos - 2018. Secretaría Técnica de Planificación, 2019. URL: https://www.dgeec.gov.py/Publicaciones/Biblioteca/POBREZA-MONETARIA%20-2018/Pobreza%20Monetaria_Boletin.pdf [Spanish].

[32] Secretaría Nacional de la Vivienda y el Hábitat (SENAVITAT), Cities Alliance, Centro de Investigación, Desarrollo e Innovación. Política Nacional de la Vivienda y el Hábitat del Paraguay [Internet]. Secretaría Nacional de la Vivienda y el Hábitat

(SENAVITAT), 2018. URL: https://www.muvh.gov.py/sitio/wp-content/uploads/2018/07/PNVH-Digital.pdf [Spanish].

[33] Cuevas ME, Aguilar ML, Elías N, Sánchez B, Irala A. Modelo de atención integral del desarrollo infantil temprano - MAIDIT. Ministerio de Salud Pública y Bienestar Social, 2016. [Spanish].

[34] Gabinete Social de la Presidencia de la República del Paraguay. Punto de partida 2019 - Sistema de Protección Social (SPS): Metas Programáticas asociadas al SPS Ejercicio Fiscal 2019 [Internet]. Gabinete Social de la Presidencia de la República del Paraguay, 2019:66. URL: https://www.gabinetesocial.gov.py/archivos/documentos/punto-partida_idi0ydzj.pdf [Spanish].

[35] Aulicino C, Díaz Langou G. Agenda de acción para la región de América Latina: Resultados del Taller "Construyendo una agenda regional para el desarrollo en la primera infancia," realizado del 14 al 16 de septiembre de 2015 en San Pablo, Brasil. International Development Bank, 2015. URL: http://1m1nttzpbhl3wbhhgahbu4ix.wpengine.netdna-cdn.com/wp-content/uploads/2016/03/FINAL-Agenda-desarrollo-integral-primera-infancia-1.pdf.

[36] Verdisco A, Cueto S, Thompson J, Neuschmidt O. PRIDI. Urgencia y Posibilidad.pdf. Banco Interamericano de Desarrollo, 2015. URL: https://publications.iadb.org/bitstream/handle/11319/6849/PRIDI.%20Urgencia%20y%20Posibilidad.pdf?sequence=4&isAllowed=y.

[37] Navarro-Cruz GE, Luschei T. International evidence on effective early childhood care and education programs: A review of best practices. Global Educ 2018;5(2):8–27.

[38] Vegas E, Santibáñez L. The promise of early childhood development in Latin America and the Caribbean. Washington, DC: World Bank, 2010.

In: Child Environmental Health Disparities ISBN: 978-1-53617-823-4
Editors: IL Rubin and J Merrick

Chapter 4

THE DEVELOPMENT OF A PRENATAL CARE HEALTH LITERACY INSTRUMENT FOR AMERICAN INDIAN MOTHERS

***Jordyn A Gunville*[1,2,3,*]**
and Jessica A Williams*[1,3], *PhD
[1]Center for American Indian Community Health
[2]Department of Family Medicine and Community Health
[3]Department of Population Health,
University of Kansas Medical Center, Kansas City,
Kansas, United States of America

ABSTRACT

American Indian (AI) women are nearly four times as likely as white women to experienced delayed prenatal care until the third trimester. Additionally, AI are the only racial/ethnic group that has not had a decline in infant mortality between 2005 and 2014. While these inequities are apparent, little is known about health literacy among AI women of

* Correspondening Author's Email: gunville@kumc.edu.

childbearing age. Existing health literacy instruments do not take the cultural context surrounding the prenatal period into account. Method: After a comprehensive review of the literature of health literacy tools and questionnaires, a measure of prenatal care health literacy for AI mothers was developed with four domains. Measure development was iterative. Cognitive interviews, a standard technique to assist validation, were used to verify the face validity of the instrument and to check understanding in the population of interest. Results: The initial instrument had 60 questions. Iterative review by experts in population health and AI health disparity research eliminated 30 duplicative questions. Cognitive interviews were conducted with AI researchers and community members, after which 5 more questions were eliminated. These interviews also help establish the validity of the tool, understanding of the questions, and suggestions for formatting of the instruments. The final instrument consists of 25 questions. Discussion: Health literacy is the ability to obtain, process, and understand health information to make knowledgeable health decisions. There is little information on health literacy specific to prenatal care and infant health among AI. This instrument was developed specifically for this marginalized population.

Introduction

American Indian infants are 2.5 times more likely to die before their first birthday than non-Hispanic White infants (1-4). While trends in maternal and infant health have been improving overall, American Indians are the only racial/ethnic group that did *not* have a decline in infant mortality between 2005 and 2014 (5). High American Indian infant mortality rates persist, despite national, tribal, and community efforts to eliminate these disparities. The American Indian infant mortality rate is 9.4 per 1,000 live births compared with a non-Hispanic White infant mortality rate of 4.9 per 1,000 live births(1). The leading causes of death for American Indian infants include congenital malformations, low birth weight, sudden infant death syndrome, and unintentional injuries (4, 6). These high rates can be attributed to confounding factors of complex interactions of behavioral, social, genetic, environmental, geographic location, economic, and heath care access (4, 7, 8).

The geographic isolation of American Indian reservations impacts the quality of life for the population, due to limited access to resources and services (8). The American Indian population is additionally impacted by harsh environmental conditions, such as uncontrollable seasonal weather, poor road conditions, and inadequate housing (9). American Indians living on reservations, whether in rural and urban areas, tend to have housing shortages, one aspect that contributes to having multiple families in one household, and poverty is also a continuing problem (10, 11).

American Indian mothers living on a reservation have additional barriers to medical care including limited insurance outside of the Indian Health Service (IHS) and limited access to transportation (12). Some reservation IHS facilities do not have the capacity to deliver infants, so if a complication arises, a pregnant mother may need to travel 2-4 hours from the reservation to deliver the infant at a better equipped hospital. Often, continuity of care is lost when entering a new health system (8).

The rate of participation for American Indian/Alaska Native women in prenatal care is significantly lower (67%) than all other races in the US (81%), at least among those women using IHS (5). In 2014, American Indian/Alaska Native mothers were 2.5 times as likely to receive late or no prenatal care as compared to non-Hispanic White mothers (13). Prenatal care rates among American Indian women who do not use IHS are unknown—another serious gap in our understanding of this complex disparity. It is important to note that the mother may start prenatal care in an IHS clinic and at the time of the delivery must go to an outside health system. This transfer to a facility outside IHS is conflicting and complicated because of the universal coverage the mother gets within the IHS health system. IHS is a health system rather than an insurance plan and federally recognized enrolled tribal members do not pay premiums or co-pays. Non-IHS providers may be paid by IHS for care given to American Indians enrolled in a federally recognized tribe—making some care appear like traditional health insurance. IHS is budgeted on a global level, meaning that all care delivered by IHS and paid for by IHS must fall within a pre-set budget that is approved annually by Congress. This is unlike most of the rest of the health system in the US, which requires insurance with patients paying premiums and copays (14). When women go outside the IHS system to receive care, their care is very difficult to track, especially if it is not eventually paid for by IHS.

Existing studies suggest that good health literacy among pregnant women is associated with better pregnancy outcomes (15-17). While health literacy is, in some sense, a universal concept, a culturally tailored measure is essential for American Indians given their barriers to care, historical trauma, differing birth practices, and cultural roles (18-20). The purpose of this study was to create a prenatal care health literacy measure specific to American Indian women to better understand literacy around prenatal care to improve birth outcomes and decrease infant mortality rates. Based on searches of PubMed, we are unaware of existing recent research on prenatal care health literacy among American Indian women. We expect that a Parental Care Health Literacy Instrument for American Indian mothers will help to break the cycle (see Figure 1) of high infant mortality by informing health care providers on proving impactful educational and clinical recommendation that are relative to the American Indian population.

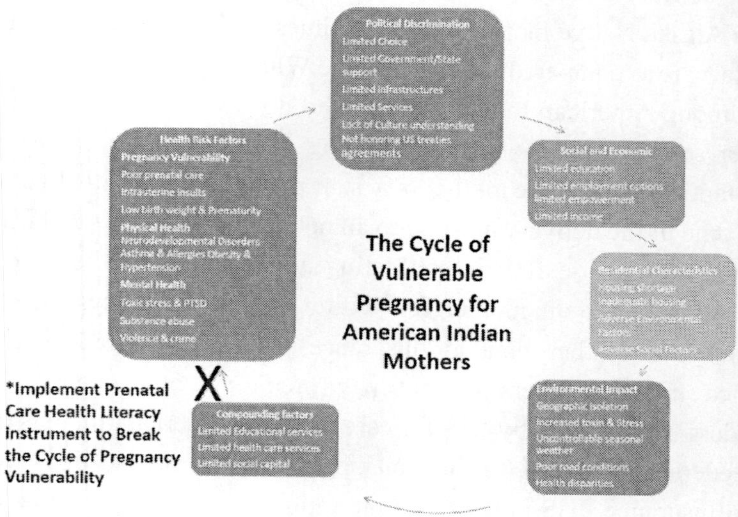

Figure 1. Conceptual model.

OUR STUDY

The development of the measure began with an assessment of existing health literacy measurement tools. A search in PubMed, Cumulative Index of Nursing and Allied Health Literature (CINAHL) and ScienceDirect was conducted to compile a list of existing health literacy tools. Content coverage and validity information were compiled for the existing tools. Additionally, educational materials that are handed out to pregnant patients from an IHS clinic located near a local university was collected. The additional information was used to further check language and content areas that are important for health education related to pregnancy. After deciding on four topic domains including: awareness (care, warning signs, symptoms), screening (when, where/how, cost), mortality (rates and ranks), and risk (activities that increase and decrease risk), questions for each domain were extracted from existing instruments to create a draft.

The draft instrument was then reviewed by three American Indian health disparity researchers and one population health expert for relevance, duplication, and content coverage for each domain. After review, certain questions were rewritten for relevance to the American Indian population.

Next, an assessment of the instrument was conducted through cognitive interviewing. Cognitive interviewing is a psychologically oriented method for empirically studying the ways in which individuals mentally process and respond to survey questionnaires (21). Cognitive interviews can be conducted for the general purpose of enhancing the understanding of how respondents carry out the task of answering survey questions. For this study cognitive interviews where used as a pretesting question and determining how they should be modified making the instrument more understandable or otherwise easier to answer.

The cognitive interviews were completed by two American Indian community members and three American Indian health disparity researchers. None of the five individuals interviewed were involved in the original draft of the instrument.

During the interview one of the study authors (JG) asked the participants to go through each question and talk about what they thought of the questions and how they processed and understood the questions. Cognitive interviews were completed to ensure that the questions had face validity and that understanding was similar across likely respondents.

FINDINGS

Two major scales measuring health literacy in the context of pregnancy were identified in the literature from the literature search described above. The first scale is a psychometrically validated measure of a woman's preferences about a future pregnancy and childbearing (Desire to Avoid Pregnancy-DAP) (22). The 14 items fit a unidimensional model, with a separation reliability of 0.90 (Cronbach's α: 0.95). The scale met established criteria for internal validity, including appropriately covering the ranges of women's preferences and correspondence between each item's response categories and overall scale scores. There was no important differential item functioning by key sociodemographic characteristics, garnering evidence for external validity (22). The second scale, the Parental Understanding of Infant Health Information: Health Literacy, Numeracy, and the Parental Health Literacy Activities Test (PHLAT), which is used to assess parental health literacy and numeracy skills in understanding instructions for caring for young children (23). During the validation of this scale, the authors found that many parents do not understand common health information required to care for their infants. The PHLAT long form and PHLAT-10 short form have good reliability and validity and may be useful tools for identifying parents who need better communication of health-related instructions (23).

After reviewing the two instruments just discussed, the authors created the original draft instrument to measure prenatal health literacy among American Indian women; it was made up of 60 questions. After review by experts in American Indian health disparity, many questions were eliminated because they were either duplicative or misleading, creating a draft long form of 30 questions. The instrument has four domains including: risk (ways to increase and decrease risk), incidence and mortality (rates and ranks), awareness (care, warning signs, symptoms), and screening (when, where/how, cost). The four domains were chosen based on health outcomes and risk factors among this marginalized population and were agreed upon jointly by three American Indian health disparity researchers who work at the Center for American Indian Community Health at the University of Kansas Medical Center and one population health expert from the Department of Population Health at the University of Kansas Medical Center (JW).

Current health care related readability formulas were used to ensure the understanding of written information in clinical and health care settings (24). We used two readability formulas, Simple Measure of Gobbledygook (SMOG) Readability formula and FRY readability formula named after developer Edward Fry. The SMOG Readability Formula is a simple method you can use to determine the reading level of your written materials. The FRY graph readability formula is used to determine the interpretation of graphics and numbers. The FRY formula is often used to provide a common standard by which the readability of documents can be measured. The instrument also includes aspects of prose (reading and writing), document (understanding and being able to fill out forms or charts/graphs), and quantitative (math, understanding numbers) literacy into the instrument; ensuring holistic representation of health literacy (25).

Each cognitive interview was around 30 to 45 minutes long and was conducted in-person. The interviewees read each question out loud, after reading the question they described their overall perception of the question including difficulty and readability. Through this interview and feedback, five additional questions were eliminated from the 30-question long form, making the final form 25 questions (see Figure 2).

Modifications of the instruments format was made based off the feedback from the cognitive interviews. If a question had fill in the blank questions, we put a number before the blank spot, making the longer fill-in-the-blank passages easier to follow.

Risk

According to the Centers for Disease Control and Prevention, birth defect occurs in the first 3 (1) _________ of pregnancy, when the organs of the baby are forming. However, some birth defects occur later in pregnancy. During the last (2) _______ months of pregnancy, the tissues and organs (3) __________ growing and developing.

Alcohol in the mother's blood passes to the baby through the (4) ___________. Drinking alcohol during pregnancy can cause miscarriage, stillbirth, and a range of lifelong physical, behavioral, and intellectual disabilities. These disabilities are known as (5) _________.

Toxoplasmosis is a common (6) __________ caused by a parasite that, when contracted by a pregnant woman, can pose serious risks to her unborn baby. To avoid, it is recommended that you do not empty cat litter from outdoor cats, wear gloves when working in the garden, do not eat undercooked (7) ________ and wash produce before consumption.

(8) Breastfeeding has been shown to decrease the risk of breast cancer.

(9) Having your child at an early age (under age 35) has been shown to increase the risk of birth defects.

(10) Smoking is also associated with lower IQ, higher miscarriage rate, higher risk of infant death at term and sudden infant death syndrome (SIDS).

(11) A miscarriage is often caused by an abnormality with the pregnancy and a result of women's activities or stresses.

(12) Smoking affects pregnant women by increasing risk for things such as preterm delivery, stillbirth, low birth weight, and ________.

(13) Nasal congestion and nose bleeds are common throughout pregnancy. They are caused by _______.

Incidence and Mortality

Use the graph below to answer questions 14-15.

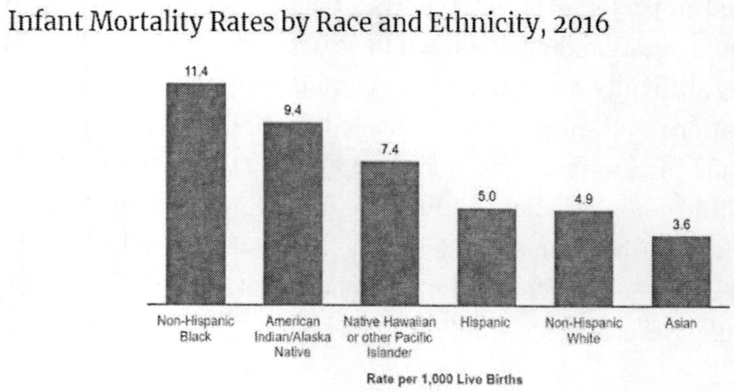

Incidence and Mortality, continued.

(14) In 2016, the infant mortality rate for American Indian/Alaska Natives was ____ per 1,000 live births.

(15) In 2016, the infant mortality rate was the highest for ____________.

Awareness

(16) Signs of miscarriage are usually vaginal bleeding and cramping.

(17) When you are pregnant, you need about 300 calories more a day than you usually eat.

(18) During pregnancy, you should continue routine dental care including cleanings, extractions, root canal, radiographs, and fillings.

(19) The increase hormones of pregnancy make the gums more susceptible to plaque buildup and bacteria causing pregnancy ____________.

Screening

(20) A preconception care visit can help women take steps toward a healthy pregnancy before they even get pregnant.

Prenatal care is the regular visits you will have with your physician during your pregnancy. In the beginning of your pregnancy, you will be seen monthly if everything is progressing well. Starting around week 28, your visits will change to every (21) _________, and then every (22) _________ the last month.

Taking folic acid daily reduces the risk for neural tube defects by (23) ________.

Most prenatal vitamins contain the recommended (24) __________ of folic acid as well as other vitamins that pregnant women and their developing fetus need.

(25) It is important to notify your doctor if your baby has not moved ten times in two hours, you have not felt the baby move all day (12 hours) or you notice a significant change in your baby's activity.

Figure 2. Final questions for prenatal health literacy instrument.

Similarly, further refinement of the instrument was made based on feedback and results from the cognitive interviews, changing wording where appropriate and arranging the instrument in chronological order from preconception to birth. The first section contains 13 questions that gage knowledge of health, prevention, and risk factors during pregnancy. The second section contains a graph showing infant mortality across race and ethnicity, two questions are based on the graph. The purpose of this section is to understand how the participants interpret information from graphics. The third section, warning signs included four true and false question asking about warning signs during pregnancy. The fourth section includes six questions in the form of multiple choice, reading passages, and true and false questions focusing on development, health, and screening points for the fetus.

Discussion

Infant mortality among American Indians is higher than among whites and is not dropping at the rate seen in other populations (1-4). While the complex interactions between risk factors such as poverty, housing, and healthcare access are central to reducing infant mortality, adequate prenatal care may address some risk factors directly (4, 9, 18). American Indian infants are nearly 4 times as likely as non-Hispanic White infants to have mothers who only received prenatal care in the third trimester, or not at all (26). Prenatal care and health screenings can improve health outcomes for both American Indian mothers and their children by providing health education and knowledge, informing behavior change, and increasing the awareness of necessary interventions (20, 27, 28).

The cycle that creates these poor outcomes can be broken. There are several intervention points. However, due to cultural differences, geographic barriers to access, differences in health policies, and legacy of discrimination, a highly interconnected approach is needed to address the high infant mortality rates among American Indians. (20, 27, 28). Prenatal health literacy among American Indian mothers has not been measured. We developed a measure of health literacy that is specific to this population to support futher efforts in the area.

This measure of prenatal health literacy is a beginning to understanding the needs and desires of this important population. Improving outcomes will only be impactful if the interventions and approaches address the literacy of the population as well as the unique factors affecting outcomes. The Prenatal Care Health Literacy Instrument breaks the cycle of childhood health disparity by improving birth outcomes at the start of pregnancy. This instrument is a tool used to assess the literacy level of the mother to enable her to get the care and information she needs during and after their pregnancy. This instrument also breaks the cycle by providing detail about health literacy in this population.

This instrument is different than other measures both in content and form. It was developed for a specific marginalized population, American Indians. American Indians have their own sovereignty, because of this, policy within different tribal nations and communities may be different than the surrounding areas. Medical training often neglects to cover this special population. Without an understanding of the cultural and contemporary life of tribal nations, as well as their traditional health practices, it is difficult for providers to form bonds with American Indian patients and have barrier-free communication. Future work will use this instrument to understand prenatal care health literacy of American Indian mothers. By understanding the health literacy of prenatal care, the gap can be closed through informing providers on what type of health information is most beneficial for American Indians mother during a prenatal care visit. This may also help bridge the gap between patients and providers, which will 'break the cycle' and improving the care for American Indian mother and reduce poor birth outcomes.

CONCLUSION

Although trends in maternal and infant health have been improving overall, American Indians are the only racial/ethnic group that did not have a decline in infant mortality (5). The high rates of infant mortality are possibly related to poor health literacy and lack of access. The development of this prenatal care health literacy instrument for American Indian mothers is a tool to evaluate prenatal care health literacy. We hope that this instrument will be used to assess health literacy so that it can be improved. Increased health literacy has the potential to improve pregnancy and birth outcomes. The next steps include, pilot research of this instrument will be conducted in American Indian communities throughout the US, both on reservations and in rural areas to assess both validity and feasibility.

References

[1] Center for Disease Control and Prevention. Infant mortality rates by race and ethnicity, 2016 URL: https://www.cdc.gov/reproductivehealth/maternalinfanthealth/infantmortality.htm.

[2] Tomashek KM, Qin C, Hsia J, Iyasu S, Barfield WD, Flowers LM. Infant mortality trends and differences between American Indian/Alaska Native infants and white infants in the United States, 1989-1991 and 1998-2000. Am J Public Health 2006;96(12):2222-7.

[3] Nakamura RM, King R, Kimball EH, Oye RK, Helgerson SD. Excess infant mortality in an American Indian population, 1940 to 1990. JAMA 1991;266(16):2244-8.

[4] Truschel L, Novoa C. American Indian and Alaska Native maternal and infant mortality: Challenges and Opportunities Center for American Progress, 2018. URL: https://www.americanprogress.org/issues/early-childhood/news/2018/07/09/451344/american-indian-alaska-native-maternal-infant-mortality-challenges-opportunities/.

[5] Infant mortality and American Indians/Alaska natives, 2015 URL: https://minorityhealth.hhs.gov/omh/browse.aspx?lvl=4&lvlid=38.

[6] US Department of Health and Human Services Office of Minority Health. Infant deaths and mortality rates for the top 4 leading cause of death for American Indian/Alaska Native 2013. URL: https://minorityhealth.hhs.gov/omh/browse.aspx?lvl=4&lvlid=38.

[7] Spencer N. The effect of income inequality and macro-level social policy on infant mortality and low birthweight in developed countries: A preliminary systematic review. Child Care Health Dev 2004;30(6):699-709.

[8] King M, Smith A, Gracey M. Indigenous health part 2: The underlying causes of the health gap. Lancet 2009;374(9683):76-85.

[9] Ludwig. T. The hidden housing crisis in Indian country. Huffpost 2013 Jul 02.

[10] Almond D, Hoynes HW, Schanzenbach DW. Inside the war on poverty: The impact of food stamps on birth outcomes. Rev Econ Statistics 2011;93(2):387-403.

[11] Wood D. Effect of child and family poverty on child health in the United States. Pediatrics 2003;112(Suppl 3):707-11.

[12] Marley TL. Ambiguous jurisdiction: Governmental relationships that affect American Indian health care access. J Health Care Poor Underserved 2019;30(2):431-41.

[13] US Department of Health and Human Services, Office of Minority Health. Percentage of mothers who received late or no prenatal care, 2014 URL: https://www.minorityhealth.hhs.gov/omh/content.aspx?lvl=3&lvlID=8&ID=3038.

[14] Zuckerman S, Haley J, Roubideaux Y, Lillie-Blanton M. Health service access, use, and insurance coverage among American Indians/Alaska natives and whites: What role does the Indian Health Service play? Am J Public Health 2004;94(1):53-9.

[15] Kohan S, Ghasemi S, Dodangeh M. Associations between maternal health literacy and prenatal care and pregnancy outcome. Iran J Nurs Midwife Res 2007;12(4):146-52.

[16] Renkert S, Nutbeam D. Opportunities to improve maternal health literacy through antenatal education: an exploratory study. Health Promot Int 2001;16(4):381-8.

[17] Solhi M, Abbasi K, Azar FEF, Hosseini A. Effect of health literacy education on self-care in pregnant women: A randomized controlled clinical trial. Int J Commun Based Nurs Midwifery 2019;7(1):2.

[18] Evans-Campbell T. Historical trauma in American Indian/Native Alaska communities: A multilevel framework for exploring impacts on individuals, families, and communities. J Interpers Violence 2008;23(3):316-38.

[19] Rockwell SL. The delivery of power: Reading American Indian childbirth narratives. Am Indian Culture Res J 1995;19(3):71-85.

[20] Barrera Jr M, Castro FG, Strycker LA, Toobert DJ. Cultural adaptations of behavioral health interventions: A progress report. J Consult Clin Psychol 2013;81(2):196.

[21] Willis GB. Cognitive interviewing: A tool for improving questionnaire design: Thousand Oaks, CA: Sage, 2004.

[22] Rocca CH, Ralph LJ, Wilson M, Gould H, Foster DG. Psychometric evaluation of an instrument to measure prospective pregnancy preferences: The desire to avoid pregnancy scale. Med Care 2019;57(2):152-8.

[23] Kumar D, Sanders L, Perrin EM, Lokker N, Patterson B, Gunn V, et al. Parental understanding of infant health information: Health literacy, numeracy, and the parental health literacy activities test (PHLAT). Acad Pediatrics 2010;10(5):309-16.

[24] Ley P, Florio T. The use of readability formulas in health care. Psychol Health Med 1996;1(1):7-28.

[25] Meade CD, Smith CF. Readability formulas: Cautions and criteria. Patient Educ Couns 1991;17(2):153-8.

[26] Lia-Hoagberg B, Rode P, Skovholt CJ, Oberg CN, Berg C, Mullett S, et al. Barriers and motivators to prenatal care among low-income women. Soc Sci Med 1990;30(4):487-94.

[27] Kvigne VL, Leonardson GR, Borzelleca J, Brock E, Neff-Smith M, Welty TK. Alcohol use, injuries, and prenatal visits during three successive pregnancies among American Indian women on the Northern Plains who have children with fetal alcohol syndrome or incomplete fetal alcohol syndrome. Matern Child Health J 2008;12(Suppl 1):37-45.

[28] Headley AJ, Harrigan J. Using the pregnancy perception of risk questionnaire to assess health care literacy gaps in maternal perception of prenatal risk. J Natl Med Assoc 2009;101(10):1041-5.

In: Child Environmental Health Disparities ISBN: 978-1-53617-823-4
Editors: IL Rubin and J Merrick

Chapter 5

BREAKING THE CYCLE OF CHILDHOOD ADVERSITY THROUGH PEDIATRIC PRIMARY CARE SCREENING AND INTERVENTIONS: A PILOT STUDY

Cristian Quizhpi[1,*], MD, Karen Schetzina[1], MD, MPH, Gayatri Jaishankar[1], MD, Robert Matthew Tolliver[1], PhD, Deborah Thibeault[2], DSW, LCSW, Hakyong Gloria Kwak[1], BS, Olushola Fapo[1], MD, MPH, Jennifer Gibson[1], MD, Katie Duvall[1], MA and David Wood, MD, MPH[1]

[1]Department of Pediatrics, East Tennessee State University
[2]Department of Social Work, East Tennessee State University, ETSU College of Public Health, Johnson City, Tennessee, United States of America

* Correspondence: Cristian Quizhpi, MD, Department of Pediatrics, East Tennessee State University, Johnson City, POBox 70578, Johnson City, TN 37614, United States. Email: QUIZHPI@mail.etsu.edu.

ABSTRACT

Adverse childhood experiences (ACEs) were defined in the landmark 1998 CDC/Kaiser Permanente Study as traumatic experiences during childhood. These include any form of abuse, neglect, or household dysfunction, such as parental divorce, intra-parental violence, parental addiction, incarceration, and mental illness. ACEs have been shown to substantially contribute to serious health problems in later life, such as mental illness, addictive behaviors, obesity, cardiovascular disease, and other chronic conditions. Numerous epidemiologic studies have demonstrated that exposure to an increased number of ACEs is associated with poorer health outcomes. While ACEs affect all socioeconomic classes, there is a higher prevalence among low-income populations. Interventions that support parenting and address family, social, and economic stressors have been shown to mitigate the impact of ACEs on future health. We sought to develop a process for addressing ACEs in a pediatric primary care office with an existing integrated Behavioral Health and Resource Team. We first assessed baseline knowledge and perceptions of ACEs among a sample of our clinic providers and local parents/caregivers. Next, we developed, and pilot tested a screening, brief intervention, and referral protocol to provide parenting resources and other supportive measures that would mitigate ACEs and promote resilience in both the parents/caregivers and children. Finally, we surveyed parents/caregivers of patients to obtain their feedback on feasibility, acceptability, and appropriateness of ACEs screening. Our long-term goals are to identify effective feasible pediatric primary care approaches to addressing trauma, promoting resiliency, and breaking the cycle of trauma and health disparities.

INTRODUCTION

The term *Adverse Childhood Experiences* (ACEs) is used to describe a wide range of traumas experienced during childhood including abuse, neglect, and other stressors. The 1998 study by the Centers for Disease Control (CDC) and Kaiser Permanente assessed 10 types of ACEs: five personal — physical abuse, verbal abuse, sexual abuse, physical neglect, and emotional neglect; and five related to dysfunction in other family members: parent alcohol abuse, domestic violence against the mother, parental incarceration, parental mental illness, or the loss of a parent through divorce, death, or abandonment (1). In the seminal study published in 1998, data was collected between

1995-1997 from 17,000 Kaiser members who completed surveys on their childhood experiences and current health status and behaviors (2). This study assessed the association between the 10 ACEs and adult health outcomes including mental health (depression, suicidality), physical health (heart disease, cancer, chronic lung disease, skeletal fractures, liver disease, obesity), and health-related behaviors (alcoholism, drug abuse, smoking, high numbers of sexual partners) (2). Prior to that survey, there had been no studied association connecting early childhood adverse experiences and adult medical problems and behaviors.

In the 1998 study, the authors aggregated the reported ACEs (each counting as one point) into a total ACE score. For example, a respondent who reported experiencing physical abuse, witnessing a parent being physically abused, losing a parent to incarceration, and experiencing life with a parent who suffered from mental illness during childhood would have an ACEs score of 4. The study concluded that individuals with higher ACE scores had a higher risk of developing the above listed poor health outcomes as adults. Persons who had experienced four or more categories of childhood exposure, compared to those who had experienced none, had 4- to 12-fold increased health risks for alcoholism, drug abuse, depression, and suicide attempt; a 2- to 4-fold increase in smoking, poor self-rated health, ≥50 sexual intercourse partners, and sexually transmitted disease; and a 1.4- to 1.6-fold increase in physical inactivity and severe obesity (2). Additionally, adults with the highest number of ACEs had a life expectancy 20 years less than those with fewer ACEs (1).

Subsequent to the CDC/Kaiser study, there have been many other studies examining the relationship between ACEs and adult health. A meta-analysis of population-based studies published through 2016 included 37 studies with 23,719 participants (3). The study found strong positive associations between an ACE score of 4+ and all measured negative health outcomes, such as overweight, diabetes, problematic drug use, violence, alcohol abuse, sexual risk taking, and mental illness. Furthermore, other studies have shown that ACEs were positively associated with poor health outcomes in adolescents, such as increased rates of early sexual debut, teen pregnancy, self-harm, suicidal ideation, and suicide attempts (4).

Furthermore, studies have shown that women who report greater exposure to ACEs have a greater risk of experiencing very early sexual initiation and increased potential exposure to Human Immunodeficiency Virus and Sexually Transmitted Illnesses' (5).

Current research is starting to show that ACEs create a pathological condition called 'toxic stress' that can play a powerful role in disrupting the architecture of the developing brain, thereby negatively influencing behavioral, educational, economic, and health outcomes (6). Childhood trauma and toxic stress adversely affect and alter a child's physiologic functioning and epigenetic expression, altering the developing immunologic and hormonal systems, further impacting their emotional and cognitive systems (2). These physiological and developmental changes findings have led the American Academy of Pediatrics (AAP) to acknowledged childhood trauma and toxic stress as foundational causes of morbidity and mortality (3). In the United States, it was estimated that in 2008 the total lifetime economic burden associated with childhood trauma was approximately $124 billion. This economic burden rivals the cost of other high-profile public health problems, such as stroke and type 2 diabetes. The lasting effects of childhood trauma and toxic stress have multi-generational consequences due to the perpetuation of the Cycle of Trauma and Health Disparities.

CYCLE OF TRAUMA AND HEALTH DISPARITIES

The Cycle of Trauma and Health Disparities is based on the Break the Cycle model for children's environmental health disparities. Abuse, neglect, and household dysfunction are examples of ACEs that the patient is exposed to during the developing years (single black circle). These events have been shown to disrupt neurological and physical development, as the child's physiological response to stress becomes dysregulated. The ongoing stress leads to both hypertrophy and over activity in the amygdala and a decrease in neural connections between the limbic system and the hippocampus, which is involved in memory function, and medial prefrontal cortex, which is involved in executive functioning and decision-making (double black circle) (7). These changes in brain development and connectivity lead to impaired memory, disordered mood, and a lack of inhibitory control which can lead to maladaptive behavioral responses such as addictive behaviors or violence. In adulthood, and as parents, the maladaptive behaviors and poor mental and physical health will have a detrimental impact on their provision of a nurturing, resourceful environment for their children and increase the likelihood that their children will also experience ACEs (3), perpetuating what we are calling the "Cycle of trauma and health disparities."

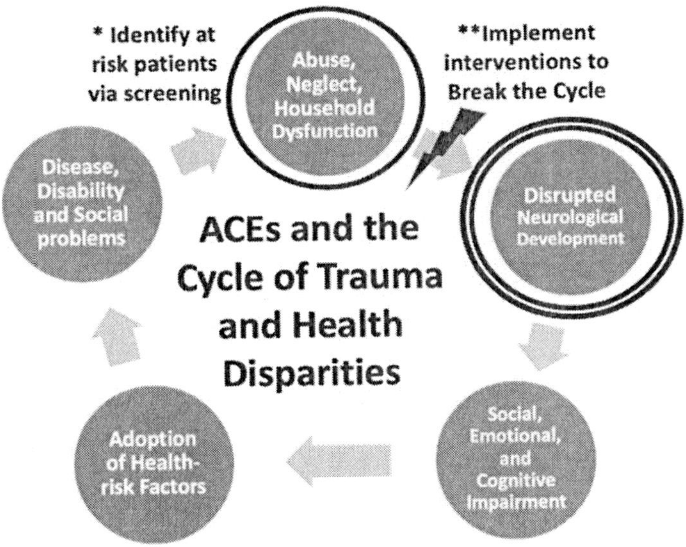

Figure 1. Cycle of trauma and health disparities.

Health care delivery systems and pediatric providers in particular, are in a unique position to identify both risk and resilience factors for the healthy development of the children and their families in their care. In response to the large and devastating burden on individual health as well as the great economic and public health burden caused by childhood trauma, the AAP issued a policy statement urging pediatricians to focus on early screening, prevention, and interventions to manage childhood trauma and toxic stress in their practices (4). However, in the primary care setting, a major stumbling block to addressing this issue is the availability of efficient ways to identify patients and families at risk for, or experiencing current trauma or the adverse effects of past childhood trauma. Moreover, there are few evidenced-based trauma-informed interventions that can be implemented in a busy primary care practice. The goal of our project was to develop a process for addressing ACEs in a pediatric primary care clinic with an existing integrated Behavioral Health and Resource team. The clinic Behavioral Health and Resource Team is led by a clinical psychologist and a clinical social worker, and consists of undergraduate and graduate level social workers, as well as doctoral level psychology students (8). The team was developed to perform assessments, brief interventions, and referrals in response to same-visit concerns identified by the pediatrician, as well as consults to address a variety of concerns (9). Research included baseline assessment of clinic provider and parent/caregiver knowledge and perceptions of ACES, development and pilot testing of an ACEs screening, brief intervention, and referral protocol, and collection of parent/caregiver feedback on screening.

The long-term goal of this work is to inform approaches for the Pediatric Primary Care Setting that will help to break the Cycle of Trauma and Health Disparities. The circled areas are those that are addressed through our screening, brief intervention, and referral program.

OUR STUDY

The setting for this study was an academic pediatric primary care clinic with an existing integrated Behavioral Health and Resource Team located in South Central Appalachia. Eighty-five percent of the children served by the clinic are publicly-insured. In order to qualify for government funded health insurance, a family of four must earn less than $34,248 per year, which is at 138% of the federal poverty line in 2018. Procedures were reviewed and approved by the East Tennessee State University Institutional Review Board.

Phase I. Knowledge of ACEs

Healthcare providers, who were not previously instructed on ACEs or ACEs screening in the clinic were invited to complete a survey on their knowledge of ACEs and their beliefs about how ACEs affect parents and children. Additionally, parents/caregivers 18 years of age or older visiting a health education table at a local community event were invited to complete the same survey. After being provided with a definition of ACEs, participants were first asked if they had heard of the term "ACEs" before. Next, using a 5-point Likert-type scale, they were asked to rate their knowledge and perceptions of how ACEs impact children's behavior, adult mental and physical health, and parenting, as well as how support systems may counteract the effects of ACEs. Responses were entered into an Excel spreadsheet and analyzed using IBM SPSS Statistics. Survey collection occurred in July 2017.

Phase II. Screening and intervention protocol development

A "Champion Team" consisting of medical, psychology, social work, nursing, case management, and community home visiting providers developed a new protocol for ACEs screening in the clinic using funding from a State of Tennessee *Building Strong Brains* grant. The team also facilitated training on ACEs and the new protocol for healthcare providers and staff in the clinic using resources from Substance Abuse and Mental Health Services Administration and Tennessee's Building Strong Brains including discussion of how to communicate about scores with families (10). The Center for Youth Wellness ACE-Questionnaire (CYW-ACE-Q) was adapted for use as a self-administered parent screener and child screener by parent/caregiver proxy (11). The CYW ACE-Q is intended for use in pediatric and family practice settings and is available in three age-specific versions and in English and Spanish. It takes approximately two to five minutes to complete the questionnaire.

Screening Questionnaire included a list of ACEs and asked the respondent to simply list the number experienced out of a possible total of ten. Due to concerns about mandatory reporting requirements, a question was added to the child screener asking the respondent to separately indicate if the following two ACEs had been experienced: "Someone pushed, grabbed, slapped, or threw something at your child OR your child was hit so hard that your child was injured or had marks," and/or "Someone touched your child's private parts or asked your child to touch their private parts in a sexual way." Screeners were distributed by the nurse during check-in for their scheduled clinic visit along with an educational resource handout on ACEs and resilience developed by the Champion Team. Education on childhood trauma and resiliency and the proposed screening protocol was provided to all clinicians and staff by the Champion Team. Parent/caregiver screeners were administered at the 1-month well child visit or first visit to the clinic. The child screeners were administered during the 12 month - 5-year annual well-child visits. Scores from the screening questionnaires were documented in the electronic health record (EHR) and discussed by the provider during the encounter. After receiving a brief summary of the clinician's concerns, also referred to as a "warm handoff," for a patient's elevated ACE scores or other behavior/social issues, the clinic Behavioral Health and Resource Team offered further assessment, resources, and support.

Families with an ACE score of 2 or higher were offered education and resources including *The Incredible Years Well Baby Program* (TIY), during well child visits in the first 9 months of life (11). TIY is designed to promote emotional and social competence and to prevent, reduce, and treat aggression and emotional problems in young children. The ultimate goal of TIY is to reduce the chance of developing later delinquent or at-risk behaviors (12). It has also been evaluated as a prevention program with children who are at risk for delinquent or high-risk behaviors because of family or demographic factors such as poverty, parental mental health problems, or poor parenting skills. The Well Baby Program was recently developed for use in the primary care setting. This program consisted of watching and discussing an age-appropriate video of parent-child interactions with a team member during the visit. A summary handout of parenting tips from the program was also provided.

Families with an ACE score of 4 or higher received education and resources from the Behavioral Health and Resource Team and were invited to participate in home or group visits including up to 10 hours of *Nurturing Parenting* (NP) (13). NP is an evidence-based program shown to improve parenting skills, problem solving, communication, and developmentally-appropriate expectations and to decrease violence in families at high risk of child maltreatment within diverse populations (13, 14).

All families seen during this period for well child visits were provided with locally-developed *ReadNPlay for a Bright Future* materials and *Reach Out and Read* books and were referred to *ReadNPlay* family community events (15). Care was coordinated for referred patients during bimonthly team conferences.

The number of patients and parents/caregivers with elevated screening results referred to the parenting programs was abstracted from the EHR on a monthly basis during the project period (October 1, 2017-June 30, 2018). Percentages were calculated based on the number of well child visits performed with screener administered during the project period.

Due to funding constraints, the local Nurturing Parenting program referral resource was discontinued during phase three.

Phase III. Parent/caregiver feedback on screening

A survey was constructed to assess parent/caregiver perceptions of acceptability, appropriateness, and feasibility of ACEs screening and interventions. The surveys were developed using the Acceptability of Intervention Measure (AIM), Intervention Appropriateness Measure (IAM), and Feasibility of Intervention Measure framework. Each construct was evaluated with four-item measures of implementation outcomes that are often considered "leading indicators" of implementation success (16). Each indicator was graded on a 1 to 5 scale, with 1 being completely disagree and

5 being completely agree using the following acceptability, appropriateness and feasibility constructs:

Our team created study flyers containing information about ACEs and ACEs scores, which were offered to parents who completed an ACE-Q screener during their child's office visit in one of three resident continuity clinics during April-May 2019. Parents who wished to complete a feedback survey did so after the visit before leaving clinic. As compensation for their time, parents were offered a small toy or book for their child at the completion of feedback survey. Survey data was entered into IBM SPSS Statistics and summarized descriptively using means, standard deviations, and percentages. A summary mean of the four items for acceptability, feasibility, and appropriateness was also calculated.

FINDINGS

During the first phase of the study, 51 parents/caregivers and 16 healthcare providers in the clinic were surveyed in Summer 2017. Results are shown in Table 1 and Figures 1 and 2. The majority of the respondents were white females within the 25-44 years age group. Fewer than one-third of parents/caregivers in this sample had heard of the term "ACEs" prior to receiving this survey. However, after being provided with a definition of ACEs, most respondents agreed that ACEs could affect children's behavior and adult mental health. Agreement was less for perceptions of effects on physical health in adults. Most respondents recognized that a parent's own ACE exposure could make parenting more difficult and that having a strong support system is helpful in counteracting these negative effects. At the start of the study, it was surprising that only half of healthcare providers were familiar with the term ACEs. After being provided with a definition of ACEs, most healthcare providers agreed that multiple ACEs can have adverse effects on children and adults.

Table 1. Demographic and baseline characteristics of study population in phase I

	Parents/Caregivers (n = 51)	**Healthcare Providers (n = 16)**
Gender		
Female	78.4%	93.8%
Male	21.6%	6.3%
Age (Years)		
18-24	5.9%	12.5%
25-34	23.5%	50%
35-44	43.1%	12.5%
45-54	11.8%	12.5%
≥55	15.7%	12.5%
Race/Ethnicity		
White	84.3%	87.5%
Hispanic/Latino	3.9%	0%
Black/African American	7.8%	0%
Asian/Pacific Islander	3.9%	12.5%
Heard of ACEs before	27.5%	50%

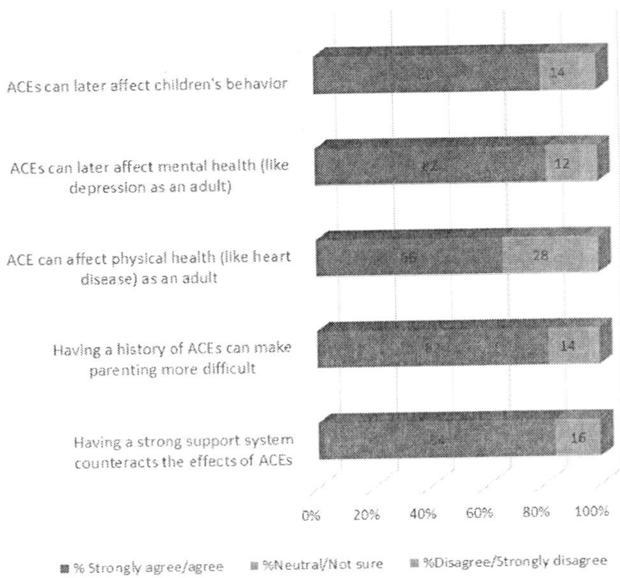

Figure 2. Knowledge and perceptions of parents/caregivers about ACEs (n = 51) Phase I.

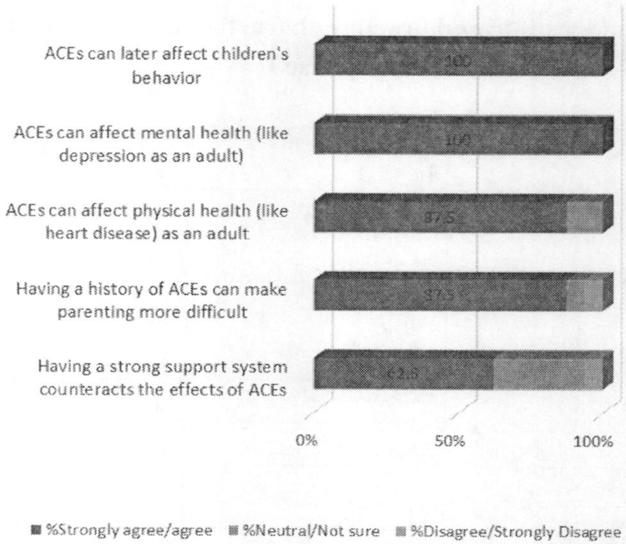

Figure 3. Knowledge and perceptions of health professionals about ACEs (n = 16): Phase I.

Table 2. Demographic characteristics of parent/caregiver ACE-Q screening feedback survey respondents during Phase III

Parent/Caregiver Demographics	# (%)
Age	
18-24 years	7 (41.2%)
25-34 years	6 (35.3%)
35-44 years	1 (5.9%)
45-54 years	2 (11.8%)
55-64 years	0
65 or older	1 (5.9%)
Race/Ethnicity	
Caucasian	15 (88.2%)
Hispanic	2 (11.8%)
Gender	
Female	13 (76.5%)
Male	4 (23.5%)

Phase II: ACEs screening and intervention protocol development and pilot-testing

Among the 96 parents/caregivers screened, 37.5% reported an ACE score of four or higher and 53.1% reported an ACE score of two or higher for themselves. Out of 66 child screeners completed for children 1-5 years of age, parents/caregivers reported ACEs score of four or higher in 3% of children. Based on our screening protocol, we referred over one third of families for Nurturing Parenting and over one half of patient families with infants 1-9 months of age for TIY.

Table 3. Means and standard deviations for acceptability, feasibility, and appropriateness items (1 = Completely Disagree; 2 = Disagree; 3 = Neutral, 4 = Agree, 5 = Completely Agree)

Question	Mean (standard deviation)
Acceptability	Possible range: 1-5
The ACE-Q screening during my office visit meets my approval	4.89 (0.323)
The ACE-Q screening during my office visit is appealing to me	4.78 (0.428)
I liked the ACE-Q screening during my office visit	4.78 (0.428)
I welcome ACE-Q screening during my office visit	4.78 (0.428)
Feasibility	Possible range 1-5
ACE-Q screening seems fitting during my child's office visit	4.72 (0.575)
ACE-Q screening seems suitable during my child's office visit	4.67 (0.594)
ACE-Q screening seems applicable during my child's office visit	4.33 (1.029)
ACE-Q screening seems like a good match for my child and my family	4.00 (1.085)
Appropriateness	Possible range: 1-5
ACE-Q screening seems implementable during my child's doctor visit	4.28 (0.826)
ACE-Q screening seems possible during my child's doctor visit	4.33 (0.907)
ACE-Q screening seems doable during my child's doctor visit	4.44 (0.784)
ACE-Q screening seems easy to use	4.67 (0.594)

A total of 18 out of 29 parents/caregivers screened for ACEs during the project period completed a feedback survey (62%). Results are shown in Tables 2 and 3. The mean summary scores for acceptability, feasibility, and appropriateness were 4.80, 4.33, and 4.43, respectively. Only two parents/caregivers completed a feedback survey on TIY, but also described it as feasible, acceptable and appropriate. The surveys filled out by both these parents shows that they marked a grade of 5 for each question on the survey provided, thus the parents strongly agreed with the intervention of the TIY. TIY was provided to only three families during the project period due to a small number of infants seen in the continuity clinics.

Discussion

In this study, we assessed the baseline knowledge and perceptions of ACEs among a sample of our clinic providers and local parents/caregivers attending the clinic with their children. We then developed and pilot tested an ACEs screening, brief intervention, and referral protocol for families with children 5 years of age and younger in a pediatric primary care clinic with an integrated Behavioral Health and Resource Team. Following implementation of the protocol, we assessed parent/caregiver feedback on ACEs screening during well child visits. ACEs screening was imperative to better understand our patient population in hope of providing those at increased risk of negative health outcomes with resources to help build resilience. In order to break the cycle of trauma and health disparities, it is imperative to identify the families experiencing trauma and to intervene as early in the life of the child as possible. Early intervention is protective against the adverse effects of toxic stress on brain development and connectivity, which can lead to impaired memory, disordered mood, and a lack of inhibitory control with regards to impulsive behavior. Thus, early intervention can be preventative against maladaptive behavioral responses such as addictive behaviors or violence (7). However, prior to our intervention, we found that less than one-third of parents/caregivers and only 50% of healthcare providers in the clinic were familiar with ACEs, suggesting a need for education among families and healthcare providers. Indeed, national data from 302 general pediatricians participating in the 2013 American Academy of Pediatrics Periodic Survey revealed that only 11% were very or somewhat familiar with the ACE study (17). Thus, our providers were found to have baseline for ACEs awareness greater than that found in a national survey. This finding is likely due to the population that our clinic serves, as 85% of our patients are publicly-insured. Nonetheless, these data suggest additional training of pediatric providers is needed to increase understanding of ACEs and long-term health outcomes.

Multiple research papers have demonstrated a graded dose-response relationship between the number of ACEs a person experienced and their health-risk behaviors (3). As the strength of the literature and evidence has grown, ACEs scores have now been linked, in the same graded dose-response relationship, to more than 40 health outcomes (18). An example particularly relevant to the Appalachia due to the opioid drug crisis, involves the graded risk increase for drug use with increasing ACEs scores. In a 2018 research paper, Tilson investigated opioid use and ACEs within the population of North Carolina and found that each ACE increased the likelihood for early initiation of drug use by 2- to 4-fold (19). Compared with people with no ACEs, people with > or = 5 ACEs were 7- to 10-fold more likely to report drug use problems, addiction, and parenteral drug use (19). These alarming findings highlight the importance of mitigating the effects of ACEs, and the need for sufficient resources to assist families with high ACE scores and is also a pre-requisite for an effective screening program. We found that the prevalence of ACEs was high in our clinic population with ACE scores of four or higher reported for 37.5% of the parents and 3% of children. An ACE score of two or higher was reported for 53.1% of parents/caregivers. Based on our screening protocol, we referred over one third of families for Nurturing Parenting and over one half of patient families for the IY. Maintaining sufficient resources to meet these needs was a challenge, and funding for Nurturing Parenting was lost during the project period. At the same time, our findings identified a large number of at-risk families, suggesting that development of additional resources should be a priority, for local community clinics such as ours to the state and federal government. The direct cost childhood trauma is measured in the billions, and the downstream effects of improved screening and propriate and adequate interventions for those affected, has the potential to decrease the rates high cost high burden disease such as obesity, heart disease and diabetes.

Notably, the rate of reported ACEs in our clinic was higher than that found in Tennessee or nationally. In 2014 in Tennessee, 17% of adults reported having experienced four or more ACEs while 42% reported two or more (20). The high percentage of ACEs among patients and parents/caregivers in our clinic was not unexpected due to the relatively low socio-economic status of our clinic population and the high rates of maternal opioid use disorder and neonatal abstinence syndrome in Northeast Tennessee (21, 22). Recent Behavioral Risk Factor Surveillance System (BRFSS) ACE data from 2011-2014 showed that nationally, 15.8% of adults reported 4 or more ACEs, and 38% reported an ACE score of 2 or more (20). Estimating the magnitude of families affected by ACEs in a pediatric primary care practice can aid in the development and allocation of services and resources.

The ACE-Q screener used in Phase II was suitable for our study population as most parents/caregivers who completed the feedback survey reported the screening as appropriate, feasible, and acceptable to them as part of a well-child visit. Providers in our clinic received training on ACEs prior to initiating screening, including on how to discuss scores with families with sensitivity, and our clinic was equipped with a Behavioral Health and Resource Team to provide support to families experiencing ACEs. Similarly, a study published in 2018 using thematic interviews with parents of children under 6 years of age attending an urban pediatric clinic found consistent support for ACEs screening for the purpose of linking to services as well as recognition of the intergenerational nature of ACEs (23). Surveys conducted with 152 predominantly Latino adults attending a federally qualified health center found that, following screening, 86% of respondents were comfortable with ACEs screening (24). In larger study of 480 pregnant women screened at 14-23 weeks gestation, over 90% were somewhat or very comfortable completing screeners and discussing results with their physician

(24). Eighty five percent somewhat or strongly agreed that clinicians should ask prenatal patients about their ACEs (25).

The American Academy of Pediatrics published a policy statement on Toxic Stress, much of which is a result of ACEs (6). Among their set of recommendations for pediatric practices was to institute screening of families at high risk for ACEs and Toxic Stress and then to provide targeted support for the parents and other caregivers by addressing key social and economic stressors through targeted referrals and by enhancing the caretakers' parenting competence (6). A potential barrier to ACEs screening is the burden on families and clinic staff at well-child visits. To address this barrier, electronic screening tools can be sent to families via email before the clinic visit. Allowing a family to fill out some of the screeners before they come to the clinic may save time during the visit and reduce the burden on families and staff. However, complete follow up of families with positive screening results reported prior to the visit may be challenging in populations with high "no-show" rates for visits, meaning the patient does not attend their recommended well child visits. Effective screening and intervention often require partnership with external agencies such as early intervention and other social services. In our practice, children have access to a Behavioral Health Resource team which includes a child psychologist and a social worker, who work in close partnerships with local social services such as Tennessee Early Intervention Services, Youth Village, and multiple behavioral therapists. However, most outpatient pediatrics clinics do not have a Behavioral Health Resource team, which can make it more challenging to access local resources or simply are situated in a region that does not have these providers. The lack of availability of expertise and partnerships with community resources to address ACEs is another potential barrier to primary care screening. Integrating professionals who can provide behavioral health and social services into primary care offices can address this barrier and improve access to needed services and resources.

In this project, we were able to initiate an ACEs screening protocol for a pediatric primary care clinic, which enabled identification of at-risk families. ACEs screening was positively perceived by most parents/caregivers. Approaches to addressing childhood trauma and considerations for ACEs screening in primary care setting has been discussed elsewhere in depth (4, 5, 8, 9). Our experience suggests that identifying provider training needs, considering parent/caregiver perceptions and preferences, and assessing resource needs are helpful initial steps. The presence of integrated behavioral health and social services in a clinic setting can be invaluable in addressing the needs of families at-risk for experiencing challenges because of their ACE score.

Conclusion

Given the high prevalence of ACEs and toxic stress and the high burden of down-stream physical and mental health problems related to these exposures, it is imperative to continue to explore optimal approaches for primary care practices to integrate screening protocols to identify families at risk, to develop sensitive and skilled staff to assist families, and to build partnerships with community organizations that can help support families, prevent ACEs, and break the cycle of trauma and health disparities.

References

[1] Larkin H, Shields JJ, Anda RF. The health and social consequences of adverse childhood experiences (ACE) across the lifespan: an introduction to prevention and intervention in the community. External J Prev Interv Community 2012;40(4):263-70.

[2] Felitti VJ, Anda RF, Nordenberg D, Williamson DF, Spitz AM, Edwards V, Koss MP, Marks JS. Relationship of childhood abuse and household dysfunction to many of the leading causes of death in adults. The Adverse Childhood Experiences (ACE) Study. Am J Prev Med 1998;14(4):245-58.

[3] Hughes K, Bellis MA, Hardcastle KA, Sethi D, Butchart A, Mikton C, et al. The effect of multiple adverse childhood experiences on health: A systematic review and meta-analysis. Lancet Public Health 2017;2(8):e356-66.

[4] Forkey H, Conn AM. Childhood Trauma Management in Primary Care. Adv Pediatr 2018;65(1):143-58.

[5] Tsuyuki K, Al-Alusi NA, Campbell JC, Murry D, Cimino AN, et al. Adverse childhood experiences (ACEs) are associated with forced and very early sexual

initiation among Black women accessing publicly funded STD clinics in Baltimore, MD. PLoS One 2019;14(5):e0216279.

[6] Garner, AS, Shonkoff JP, Siegel BJ, Dobbins MI, Earls MI, McGuinn L, et al. Early childhood adversity, toxic stress, and the role of the pediatrician: Translating developmental science into lifelong health. Pediatrics 2012;129;e224;.

[7] Shonkoff JP, Boyce WT, McEwen BS. Neuroscience, molecular biology, and the childhood roots of health disparities: building a new framework for health promotion and disease prevention. JAMA 2009;301(21):2252-9.

[8] Polaha J, Schetzina, KE, Baker, K. A collaborative practice training model for pediatric primary care. Int J Health Sci Educ 2016;3(2):1-10.

[9] Polaha J, Schetzina KE, Baker K, Morelen D. Adoption and reach of behavioral health services for behavior problems in pediatric primary care. *Fam Systems Health 2018;36*(4):507-12.

[10] SAMHSA-HRSA Center for Integrated Health Solutions. Trauma. URL: https://www.integration.samhsa.gov/clinical-practice/trauma.

[11] Center for Youth Wellness ACE-Questionnaire (CYW ACE-Q Child, Teen, Teen SR). San Francisco, CA: Center for Youth Wellness.

[12] Pontoppidan M, Klest SK, Sandoy TM. The Incredible Years Parents and Babies Program: A pilot randomized controlled trial. PLoS One 2016;11(12):e0167592.

[13] Family Development Resources. Nurturing parenting programs and over 30 years of evidence. URL: http://nurturingparenting.com/nppsevidence.html

[14] Collins CL, Fetsch RJ. A review and critique of 16 major parent education programs. J Extension 2012;50(4):1-25.

[15] National Resource Center for Patient/Family-Centered Medical Home. ReadNPlay for a bright future. URL: https://medicalhomeinfo.aap.org/practices/Pages/ReadNPlay-for-a-Bright-Future.aspx.

[16] Weiner BJ, Lewis CC, Stanick C, Powell BJ, Dorsey CN, Clary AS, et al. Psychometric assessment of three newly developed implementation outcome measures. Implement Sci 2017;12(1):108.

[17] Kerker BD, Storfer-Isser A, Szilagyi M, Stein RE, Garner AS, O'Connor KG, et al. Do Pediatricians Ask About Adverse Childhood Experiences in Pediatric Primary Care. Acad Pediatr 2016;16(2):154-60.

[18] Dube S, Felitti V, Dong M, Chapman D, Giles W, Anda R. Childhood abuse, neglect, and household dysfunction and the risk of illicit drug use: The adverse childhood experiences study. Pediatrics 2003;111(3):564-72.

[19] Tilson EC. Adverse childhood experiences (ACEs): An important element of a comprehensive approach to the opioid crisis. NC Med J 2018;79(3):166-9.

[20] Merrick MT, Ford DC, Ports KA, Guinn AS. Prevalence of adverse childhood experiences from the 2011-2014 behavioral risk factor surveillance system in 23 States. JAMA Pediatrics 2018;172(11):1038-44.

[21] Miller AM and McDonald M. Tennessee Department of Health Neonatal Abstinence Syndrome Surveillance Annual Report 2018. URL: https://www.tn.gov/content/dam/tn/health/documents/nas/NAS%20Annual%20Report%202018%20FINAL.pdf.

[22] Agarwal P, Wood D. Factors affecting the length of Stay in drug exposed infants admitted to the neonatal intensive care unit. Int Public Health J 2018;10(3):265-74.

[23] Conn AM, Szilagyi MA, Jee SH, Manly JT, Briggs R, Szilagyi, PG. Parental perspectives of screening for adverse childhood experiences in pediatric primary care. Fam Syst Health 2018;36(1):62-72.

[24] Goldstein E, Athale N, Sciolla A, Catz, S, Patient preferences for discussing childhood trauma in primary care. Perm J 2017;21:16-55.

[25] Flanagan T, Alabaster A, McCaw B, Stoller N, Watson C, Young-Wolff KC. Feasibility and acceptability of screening for adverse childhood experiences in prenatal care. J Women's Health 2018;27(7):903-11.

In: Child Environmental Health Disparities ISBN: 978-1-53617-823-4
Editors: IL Rubin and J Merrick

Chapter 6

EDUCATING CLINIC SUPPORT STAFF TO ENHANCE EARLY LEARNING ENVIRONMENTS THROUGH PEDIATRIC WELL-CHILD VISITS

Cori Walker, Asher Liu, Snigdha Gupta, Fuad Baroody, MD and Dana Suskind*, MD
TMW Center for Early Learning and Public Health,
University of Chicago, Chicago, Illinois, United States

ABSTRACT

A rich early language environment in the first years of life is important for optimal language and cognitive development. Socioeconomic disadvantage in a child's early language environment can have long-term impacts on educational attainment, employment opportunities, and health outcomes. In an effort to enhance the early language milieu for children from low-income households, this study aims to 1) improve pediatric clinic support staff's knowledge about early cognitive and language development and 2) positively influence their perceptions of the role they can play in educating parents/caregivers about the importance of early language

* Corresponding Author's Email: dsuskind@surgery.bsd.uchicago.edu.

exposure in the first three years of life. The study was run as a quasi-experimental, One-Group, Pretest-Posttest Design. The participants were pediatric clinic support staff members from four clinics in the Chicago area (n = 58). Participants' knowledge and perceptions were assessed one week prior to a curriculum presentation intervention and immediately following the intervention. Analysis showed a significant increase in participants' knowledge of early cognitive and language development post-intervention (infancy: M = 24.74 vs. M = 28.05, P = 9.63E-09; early childhood: M = 25.78 vs. M = 29.90, P = 1.39E-11). Clinic support staff also reported that after attending the presentation, they felt more comfortable and were more likely to discuss these topics with parents/caregivers in clinic. This study highlights the importance of educating clinic staff about early language and cognitive development and informing them of the crucial role they can play in helping to enhance early language environments for their young patients, particularly those from low socioeconomic backgrounds.

INTRODUCTION

The first three years of life are said to be the most important for cognitive and language development. During this period, new neural connections are formed at a rate of over 1 million per second (1). Early social experiences and rich language interactions with nurturing caregivers are critical for this rapid brain development and set the foundation for future learning (2, 3). A child's early language environment is an important, yet often overlooked, social determinant of health (4). Research suggests that disparities in the quality of this early language environment exist and disproportionately affect those in poverty (5). These disparities have been shown to negatively impact brain growth—as well as future educational, occupational, and health outcomes—among socioeconomically disadvantaged children (6-8).

Research shows that the negative impacts of poverty on brain development become apparent well before children enroll in school. In a longitudinal study by Tamara Halle et al. (9), nine-month old infants in families of low socioeconomic status (SES) scored lower on cognitive development assessments than their peers. This disparity tripled in severity by 24 months of age. That being so, programs aimed at supporting children's cognitive development after they begin school may come too late to alter the trajectories of children's neurocognitive development. (10). Therefore, interventions in the critical first three years of life are necessary to prevent such disparities at their onset.

Parents and caregivers in the home are the key mediators of a child's early learning environment. Disparities in early social interactions and language input among children from differing SES backgrounds have been attributed to differences in parental knowledge of infant development (11, 12). Further, parental knowledge about the importance of early language exposure has been shown to be predictive of parental behaviors with their children (13). These behaviors inform the quality of adult-child interactions and a child's early language environment. This environment sets the foundation for a child's brain and language development, which sets the basis for their school readiness and educational attainment. Lower educational attainment has been shown to result in decreased employment opportunities, limited residential options, and ultimately, poor health outcomes (4). The diagram below represents this cycle of early learning disparities.

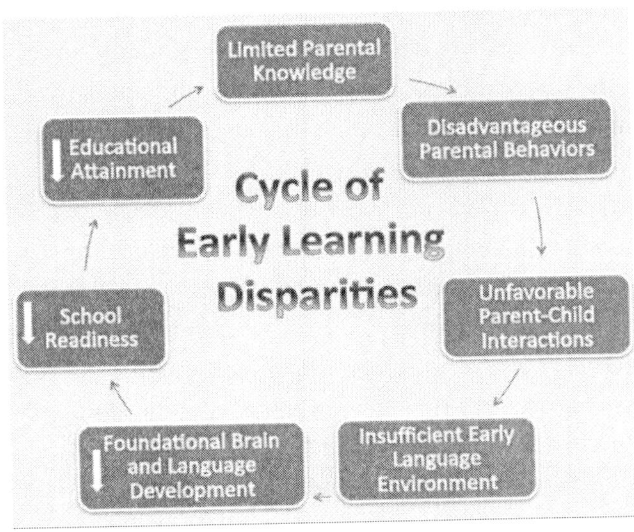

Figure 1. The cycle of early learning disparities.

Fortunately, studies have shown that well-planned, parent-directed interventions in low-income populations can significantly improve various parenting behaviors with their children (14). Therefore, interventions to empower all parents with increased knowledge of early brain development and everyday strategies to enrich their children's early language environments represent a promising opportunity to reduce educational inequities and subsequently break the cycle of early learning disparities.

There are 12 recommended routine well-child pediatric visits during the first three years of life (15). As a result, pediatricians and pediatric clinic staff are uniquely positioned to intervene during this critical period of foundational brain development. In fact, in 2017, the American Academy of Pediatrics established 'early brain and cognitive development' as an integrated child health priority in their "Agenda for children" (16). However, while studies have shown that parents want more information on early childhood learning at pediatric visits, they do not regularly receive this desired insight (17). A recent study surveying 236 parents in Chicago area clinics found that only a minority of parents reported receiving information on cognitive development topics at well-child visits, such as "brain growth" [25.8%], "how babies learn" [13.1%], and "learning to talk" [9.3%] (18).

While pediatricians are often considered the primary source of guidance for parents, they have a large mandate to cover in the relatively brief, well-child visit and may not have the time to engage families and emphasize all anticipatory guidance topics equally (19, 20). The clinical support staff can play a meaningful role in actively engaging families by providing information about language interactions and enhancing discussions of important topics during clinic visits (21). Therefore, with the objective to break the cycle of early learning disparities (see Figure 1), this study intends to use pediatric clinics - and more specifically, the support staff in these clinics - as an access point to positively impact parental knowledge of early brain development (see Figure 2). Our study aimed to create, deliver, and test a curriculum intervention designed to improve pediatric clinic support staff's knowledge about early cognitive and language development, and positively influence their perceptions of the role they can play in educating parents/caregivers about the importance of early language environments during pediatric clinic visits. We hypothesized that after attending our intervention, study participants would exhibit improved knowledge and report increased comfort and likelihood to engage in discussion of these topics with parents during well-child visits. The ultimate goal of this intervention was to see if we could cultivate a pediatric clinic culture that identifies early cognitive and language development as a priority, and considers educating parents on this topic a standard of care.

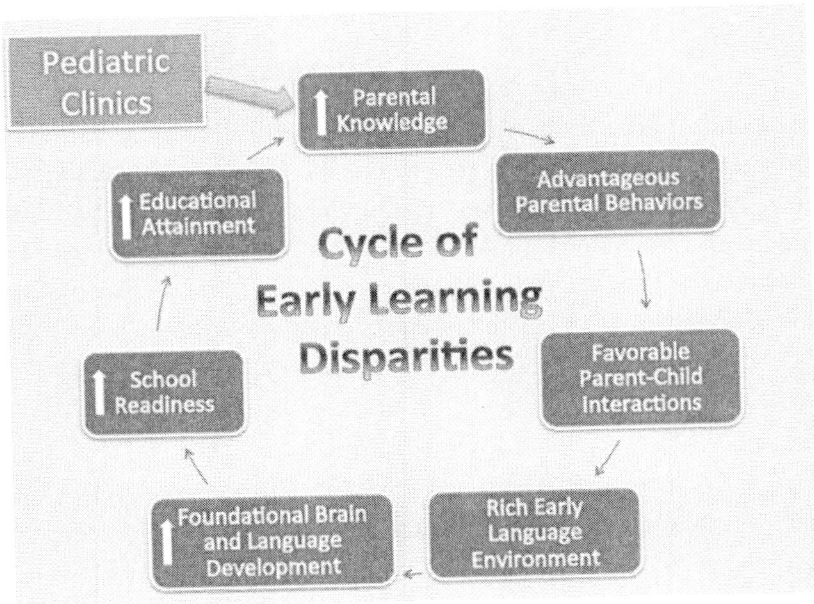

Figure 2. Use of pediatric clinics to break the cycle of early learning disparities.

OUR STUDY

This study was conducted at four pediatric clinics that serve predominantly families with public assistance in the Chicago area. The study began in December 2018 and concluded in February 2019. The clinics were identified through email correspondence with clinic coordinators or directors. All pediatric clinic staff other than the physicians (i.e., nurses, medical assistants, laboratory technicians, receptionists, etc.) were asked to volunteer to participate in the study, including attending an intervention and responding to surveys at their clinic. Staff members were eligible to participate if they were at least 18 years old and English-speaking. Participants were verbally consented prior to the curriculum intervention and received a $50 gift card as compensation. The Biological Sciences Division Institutional Review Board at the University of Chicago Medicine (IRB#12-1172-CR006) approved this study.

Intervention

A curriculum intervention was developed specifically for pediatric clinic support staff. The multimedia curriculum included an explanation of the science behind early cognitive and language development as well as common misconceptions about these topics and specific strategies and examples for addressing these topics with parents in clinic. The intervention was delivered in the form of an in-person, group presentation at each clinic.

Measures

A demographics questionnaire was administered to study participants about one week prior to the curriculum intervention. Paper versions of the questionnaires were delivered to the clinic for participants to complete at their leisure. The completed questionnaires were collected from the clinic about two days prior to the scheduled intervention date.

Knowledge

Along with the demographics questionnaire, participants completed the Scale of Parent/Provider Expectations and Knowledge (SPEAK) (22). The SPEAK assesses providers' expectations on developmental milestones and their knowledge about the role of caregiver responsiveness and inputs in children's cognitive and language development during infancy (birth-6 months) and early childhood (birth-5 years). Participants responded to 1 item on a 6-point scale, ranging from 0 (in elementary school, 6 years and up) to 5 (as an infant, 0 to 6 months), and 17 items on a 4-point scale, ranging from 0 (definitely true) to 3 (definitely not true). Two SPEAK sum scores including Infancy (a = .74) and Early Childhood (a = .72) were calculated. Higher scores represented more knowledge. This questionnaire was administered to participants a second time immediately following the curriculum intervention.

Beliefs

Participants were given qualitative questions to assess their initial beliefs about educating parents on early cognitive development and the importance of early language exposure. Multiple choice questions assessed what role the participants believed they had in educating parents and their comfort level in doing so. Post-intervention questions assessed if participants found the presentation useful and whether or not it made them feel more comfortable discussing topics such as early language and cognitive development with parents during well-child visits.

Reported behaviors

To assess baseline behaviors, a pre-intervention question asked the participants if they currently discuss early language and brain development with parents/caregivers of infants. Perceived barriers to discussing these topics with parents, along with potential solutions to these barriers, were evaluated with checklist items and free response. Post intervention, participants were asked whether or not the curriculum presentation made them more likely to discuss early language and cognitive development with parents of young children during well-child visits.

Statistical analysis

Two SPEAK score sums, i.e., infancy (birth-6 months) and early childhood (birth-5 years), for each participant were calculated from the pre- and post-intervention SPEAK surveys. Pre- and post-intervention scores were compared using two-tailed t-tests in Microsoft Excel. In order to investigate whether the intervention had similar effects on participants with varying education, we compared the baseline and post-intervention SPEAK scores among participants with high education (Bachelor's degree or above) and participants with low education (less than Bachelor's degree) separately. Responses to pre- and post-intervention qualitative questions were tallied and the percentages of each response on pre-intervention questions were compared to those from the post-intervention questions.

FINDINGS

The sample included 58 clinic staff members with a 90.6% retention rate among the 64 participants recruited originally. The majority of participants were female (86.2%) mainly in the 25-34 and 35-44 age ranges (36.2% and 25.9%, respectively; see Table 1). Most participants identified as Black or African American (46.6%), followed by English-speaking Hispanic or Latino participants of any race (27.6%, see Table 1). For education level, the majority of study participants had completed some college credit, technical training or an associate's degree, but had not obtained a bachelor's degree (60.3%; see Table 2). Participants held a variety of job titles within the clinics. The largest group was Medical Assistants (37.9%) followed by roles that involved assisting patients at the clinic's front desk (i.e., Registration, Receptionist, Referral Coordinator, Patient Service Representative; 15.5%; see Table 2). The third largest group of participants was Nurses (13.8%).

Table 1. Participant demographics

Variable		Category	% (n = 58)
Age		18-24	3.4
		25-34	36.2
		35-44	25.9
		45-54	22.4
		55-64	12.1
		65+	0
Sex		Female	86.2
		Male	8.6
		Prefer not to answer	5.2
Race	Hispanic or Latino	Any race	27.6
	Non-Hispanic	Black or African American	46.6
		White	10.3
		Asian or Pacific Islander	3.5
		Multiracial	1.7
	Prefer not to answer		10.3

Table 2. Participant education and job title

Variable	Category	% (n = 58)
Education level	High school graduate, or equivalent (GED)	8.6
	Some college credit, no degree	20.7
	Technical training	24.1
	Associate degree	15.5
	Bachelor's degree	17.2
	Postgraduate degree	12.1
	No response	1.7
Job Title	Medical Assistant	37.9
	Registration/Receptionist/Referral Coordinator/PSR	15.5
	Nurse	13.8
	Manager/Clinic Coordinator	6.9
	Lab Tech	5.2
	Social Worker/Case Manager	5.2
	Medical Interpreter	3.4
	Maintenance/Security	3.4
	Nurse Practitioner	1.7
	Lactation Specialist	1.7
	OutReach Manager	1.7
	Healthy Steps Specialist	1.7
	No response	1.7

Knowledge

There was a significant increase in Infancy SPEAK scores from baseline (M = 24.74, SD = 4.18) to post-intervention (M = 28.05, SD = 2.90; see Table 3). There was also a significant increase in Early Childhood SPEAK scores from baseline (M = 25.78, SD = 4.37) to post-intervention (M = 29.90, SD = 2.67; see Table 4). When comparing baseline and post-intervention SPEAK scores by participant education level (less than Bachelor's degree and Bachelor's degree or above), there was a significant increase in SPEAK scores from baseline to post-intervention for both education levels (see Tables 5 and 6).

Table 3. Infancy SPEAK change in knowledge

	Mean	N	SD	SE Mean	t	df	Significance
Baseline	24.74	58	4.18	.549			
Post-Intervention	28.05	58	2.90	.381	-6.711	57	9.63E-09

Table 4. Early childhood SPEAK change in knowledge

	Mean	N	SD	SE Mean	t	df	Significance
Baseline	25.78	58	4.37	.574			
Post-Intervention	29.90	58	2.67	.350	-8.418	57	1.39E-11

Table 5. Infancy SPEAK change in knowledge by education level

Education Level	Time Point	Mean	N	SD	SE Mean	t	df	Significance
Less than Bachelor's Degree	Baseline	24.70	40	4.046	0.640			
	Post-Intervention	27.98	40	3.084	0.488	-5.344	39	0.000
Bachelor's Degree or Higher	Baseline	24.94	17	4.710	1.142			
	Post-Intervention	28.18	17	2.604	0.631	-3.673	16	0.002

Table 6. Early childhood SPEAK change in knowledge by education level

Education Level	Time Point	Mean	N	SD	SE Mean	t	df	Significance
Less than Bachelor's Degree	Baseline	25.85	40	3.718	0.588			
	Post-Intervention	29.83	40	2.735	0.432	-7.493	39	0.000
Bachelor's Degree or Higher	Baseline	25.88	17	5.732	1.390			
	Post-Intervention	29.94	17	2.609	0.633	-3.833	16	0.001

Beliefs

Prior to the curriculum intervention, participants were asked to respond to the statement "In my role, I feel comfortable sharing information about children's language and brain development with parents/caregivers of infants." Responses greatly varied with 10.5% "Strongly Agree," 47.4% "Agree," 31.6% "Disagree," and 10.5% "Strongly Disagree" (N = 57). Participants were also asked to gauge what role they thought they played "in teaching parents about their child's early language and brain development.' 35% of study participants felt that they played either a "Significant" or "Moderate Role" in this, while 36.8% responded "Minor Role" and 24.6% responded "No Role" (N = 58).

After the curriculum intervention, 100% of study participants replied "Strongly Agree" or "Agree" to finding the presentation useful. 98.3% reported "Strongly Agree" or "Agree" to the statement: "The strategies presented in this curriculum make me more comfortable discussing topics such as early language and cognitive development with parents during well-child visits" (N = 58).

Reported behaviors

On the pre-intervention survey, 81% of participants answered "Never" or "Not Often" when asked if they "currently discuss early language and brain development with parents/caregivers of infants" (N = 58). "No expertise in this topic" was the most selected reason for what prevents participants from discussing these topics in their interactions with parents/caregivers. (50%; see Table 7). Participants felt that having pamphlets to provide parents (69%) and more training on the topic (65.5%) would make them more likely to talk about early language and brain development in their interactions with parents/caregivers of infants (see Table 8).

Table 7. Perceived Barriers to discussions. Some themes among free response answers from participants that selected "Other" include limited interactions with parents/patients, feeling that other professionals in clinic should have these discussions with parents, and not wanting to spread false information

What prevents you from discussing early language and brain development in your interactions with parents/caregivers of infants? (Select all that apply)	**%**
Time constraints	39.7
No expertise in this topic	50.0
More important topics to discuss with parents	1.7
Difficult topic for parents/caregivers to understand	6.9
Not a part of my job description	37.9
Other	13.8

Table 8. Reported items to increase likelihood of discussions. Free response answers from participants that selected "Other" either reiterated the need for more training on this topic or stated that having these discussions is not a part of their job description

What are some things that would make you more likely to talk about early language and brain development in your interactions with parents/caregivers of infants? (Select all that apply.)	**%**
More time	43.1
More training on the topic	65.5
Having pamphlets to provide parents	69.0
Making this an EMR checklist item to discuss	15.5
Financial incentive	8.6
Other	15.5

After attending the curriculum intervention, 100% of study participants stated that they "Agree" or "Strongly agree" with the statement: "I am more likely to discuss early language and cognitive development with parents of young children during well-child visits" (N = 58).

DISCUSSION

Rich language environments, shaped by nurturing adult-child interactions, are critical to building children's brains in the first three years of life. Disparities in early language environments exist and disproportionately affect those in poverty. Not only do these early learning disparities negatively impact children's cognitive and language development, they also have long-term impacts on educational attainment, future employment and economic security, and health outcomes. Because parents are the key mediators of a child's learning environment during this early period, impacting parental knowledge of early brain development, and consequently impacting their interactions with their children, is a pivotal step in breaking the cycle of early learning disparities. In an effort to leverage the touchpoints that well-child visits offer, this study aimed to enhance pediatric clinic support staff's knowledge about early language and cognitive development and impact their beliefs about the critical role they can play in educating parents about the importance of early interactions. The study was conducted in four pediatric clinics, and the intervention included an in-person curriculum presentation focused on the science of early brain development the role of pediatric clinic support staff, and strategies to discuss brain and language development with parents during well-child visits.

Findings of the present study demonstrate an increase in knowledge of early cognitive and language development among pediatric clinic support staff after attending the educational presentation. The study also reveals that the staff members are more willing to discuss these topics with parents when they feel properly equipped to do so. The commonly reported lack of expertise on early brain and language development, and the need for more training on this topic in order to discuss with parents, can be addressed by providing the support staff with the education they desire, as well as easy-to-implement strategies to promote these discussions with parents in clinic. The findings of our study show that the curriculum intervention we created had an immediate positive impact on knowledge of early cognitive and language development for staff members regardless of their varying levels of education.

This study demonstrates the need for providing ongoing education to the clinic support staff and supporting them with tools and strategies to engage parents. Using their unique access to families, pediatric office staff can promote the importance of early language environments and encourage families to have rich language interactions with their children. Utilizing all pediatric clinic support staff to participate in these discussions with parents and caregivers can directly enhance patient access to important information during clinic visits (23). It can also improve overall clinic efficiency and ensure providers feel well supported, and clinic support staff feel more empowered to support parents (24, 25). These discussions with parents may have immediate positive effects on the parent-child relationship, and with continued reinforcement, could potentially contribute to long-term positive educational outcomes for all children.

Limitations

Some limitations of this study should be noted. As a quasi-experimental design, our study lacks a control group and randomization. Although participants reported an increased likelihood to discuss brain and language development with parents in clinic, our study did not include any behavior measures to assess if these discussions did increase post-intervention. A longer study timeline would allow for the addition of these behavior measures and a third SPEAK assessment at a later point in time to measure for retention of the knowledge gained from our intervention. It is also not clear whether changes in clinic staff behavior would have a significant impact on child developmental outcomes, which is the ultimate goal of this effort. Future research might be able to examine this aspect more fully.

Conclusion

This study highlights a valuable opportunity for educating pediatric clinic support staff about early language and cognitive development and the important role they may play in enhancing early language environments for their patients. Providing training to pediatric clinic staff may help increase awareness of the importance of early language exposure, but further studies are needed to investigate the true impact of this intervention on the quantity and quality of discussions with parents in clinic. Leveraging the routine well-child visits and all clinic staff members to make these discussions a standard of care has the potential to help break the cycle of early learning disparities experienced by socioeconomically disadvantaged children at their earliest onset.

References

[1] Center on the Developing Child. Harvard University. Brain architecture. URL: https://developingchild.harvard.edu/science/key-concepts/brain-architecture/.

[2] Gervain J. Plasticity in early language acquisition: the effects of prenatal and early childhood experience. Curr Opin Neurobiol 2015;35:13-20.

[3] Ronfani L, Vecchi Brumatti L, Mariuz M, Tognin V, Bin M, Ferluga V, et al. The complex interaction between home environment, socioeconomic status, maternal IQ and early child neurocognitive development: a multivariate analysis of data collected in a newborn cohort study. PLoS One 2015;10:1-13.

[4] Maggi S, Irwin LJ, Siddiqi A, Hertzman C. The social determinants of early child development: an overview. J Paediatr Child Health 2010;46:627-35.

[5] LoRe D, Ladner P, Suskind D. Talk, read, sing: early language exposure as an overlooked social determinant of health. Pediatrics 2018;142:e20182007

[6] Hanson JL, Hair N, Shen DG, Shi F, Gilmore JH, Wolfe BL, et al. Family poverty affects the rate of human infant brain growth. PLoS One 2013;8:e80954.

[7] Hair NL, Hanson JL, Wolfe BL, Pollak SD. Association of child poverty, brain development, and academic achievement. JAMA Pediatr 2015;169:822-29.

[8] Schoon I, Parsons S, Rush R, Law J. Childhood language skills and adult literacy: a 29-year follow-up study. Pediatrics 2010;125:e459-66.

[9] Halle T, Forry N, Hair E, Perper K, Wandner L, Wessel J, et al. Disparities in early learning and development: lessons from the early childhood longitudinal study – birth cohort (ECLS-B). Washington, DC: Child Trends, 2009.

[10] Hart B, Risley TR. The early catastrophe: The 30 million word gap by age 3. Am Educator 2003;Spring:4-9.

[11] Rowe ML, Denmark N, Harden BJ, Stapleton LM. The role of parent education and parenting knowledge in children's language and literacy skills among white, black, and latino families. Infant Child Dev 2015;25:198-220.

[12] Rowe ML. Child-directed speech: relation to socioeconomic status, knowledge of child development and child vocabulary skill. J Child Lang 2008;35:185-205.

[13] Leung CYY, Suskind D. What parents know matters: Parental knowledge at birth predicts caregiving behaviors at 9 months. Manuscript under review.

[14] Van Mourik K, Crone MR, de Wolff MS, Reis R. Parent training programs for ethnic minorities: a meta-analysis of adaptations and effect. Prev Sci 2017;18(1):95-105.

[15] American Academy of Pediatrics. AAP schedule of well-child care visits. URL: https://www.healthychildren.org/English/family-life/health-management/Pages/Well-Child-Care-A-Check-Up-for-Success.aspx

[16] American Academy of Pediatrics. AAP agenda for children—strategic plan 2017-2018. URL: https://www.aap.org/en-us/about-the-aap/aap-facts/AAP-Agenda-for-Children-Strategic-Plan/Pages/AAP-Agenda-for-Children-Strategic-Plan.aspx.

[17] Schuster MA, Duan N, Regalado M, Klein DJ. Anticipatory guidance: What information do parents receive? what information do they want? Arch Pediatr Adolesc Med 2000;154:1191–8.

[18] Leung CYY, LoRe D, Hundertmark AC, Leffel KR, Miller K, Suskind DL. Improving education on child language and cognitive development in the primary care settings through a technology-based curriculum: a randomized controlled trial. Pediatrics 2018;142:1.

[19] Coker TR, Windon A, Moreno C, Schuster MA, Chung PJ. Well-child care clinical practice redesign for young children: a systematic review of strategies and tools. Pediatrics 2013;131(1):S5-25.

[20] Mooney K, Moreno C, Chung PJ, Elijah J, Coker TR. Well-child care clinical practice redesign at a community health center: provider and staff perspectives. J Prim Care Commun Health 2015; 5(1):19-23.

[21] Greenwood DA, Parise CA, MacAller TA, Hankins AI, Harms KR, Pratt LS, et al. Utilizing clinical support staff and electronic health records to increase tobacco use documentation and referrals to a state quitline. J Vasc Nurs 2012;30:107-11.

[22] Suskind DL, Leung CYY, Webber RJ, Hundertmark AC, Leffel KR, Suskind E. Development of the survey of parent/provider expectations and knowledge (SPEAK). First Language 2017;38:312-31

[23] Baker AN, Parsons M, Donnelly SM, Johnson L, Day J, Mervis A, et al. Improving colon cancer screening rates in primary care: a pilot study emphasising the role of the medical assistant. Qual Saf Health Care 2009;18:355-9.

[24] Jerzak J. Using empowers CMAs and nursing staff to improve team-based care. Fam Pract Manag 2019;26:17-22.

[25] Hopkins K, Sinsky CA. Team-based care: saving time and improving efficiency. Fam Pract Manag 2014;21:23-9.

In: Child Environmental Health Disparities ISBN: 978-1-53617-823-4
Editors: IL Rubin and J Merrick

Chapter 7

CONTEXTUALIZING THE SOCIAL AND STRUCTURAL CONSTRAINTS OF ACCESSING AUTISM SERVICES AMONG SINGLE BLACK FEMALE CAREGIVERS

Alice Hong and Jennifer S Singh*, PhD
Georgia Institute of Technology, School of History and Sociology,
Atlanta, Georgia, United States of America

ABSTRACT

Autism spectrum disorder (ASD) affects 1 in 59 children and represent the fastest growing developmental disorder in the United States. However, disparities in ASD evaluation, diagnosis, and services exist based on social factors such as race, ethnicity, and socioeconomic status. To date, limited qualitative research has been conducted that focuses on the experiences of single black female caregivers of children with ASD who live in low-income, minority, and underserved communities in the United States. Objective: This study aimed to understand interrelated social and structural

---

* Address correspondence to: jennifer.singh@hsoc.gatech.edu.

factors that place children and their families with limited resources at risk of delayed ASD diagnostic services and limited therapeutic services. Methods: The study design is based on in-depth interviews conducted with single black female caregivers of children with ASD who rely on state Medicaid health insurance in metro Atlanta, Georgia (N = 21). A grounded theory analysis of the interviews was used to systematically identify themes and multi-level barriers to ASD services. Results: Despite improvements over the past several decades in diagnosing children with ASD, this study identified multiple and interacting social, economic, and residential barriers to accessing ASD services. Two themes were identified that contextualize barriers to ASD services: bureaucratic processes and geographic location of services. These barriers were compounded by the consequences of being a single female parent, including having limited income, employment options, and social capital. Practical recommendations to break the cycle of ASD service disparities are discussed.

Introduction

Autism spectrum disorder (ASD) is defined by the American Psychiatric Association as a lifelong neurodevelopmental disorder characterized by persistent challenges in "social communication and social interaction," and "restricted, repetitive patterns of behavior, interests, or activities" (1). According to the Centers for Disease Control and Prevention (CDC), ASD affects 1 in 59 children and is the fastest growing developmental disorder in the United States (2). Recommended treatment for ASD consists of early intensive behavioral and educational interventions (3). A trained clinician can reliably diagnose ASD in children as early as 2 years old or younger, but most children are not diagnosed with ASD until after age 4 years (2).

ASD is prevalent in all racial and ethnic groups and across all socioeconomic levels; however, disparities exist in the prevalence of ASD associated with social factors, such as by age, sex, race, ethnicity, and geographic area (2). For example, boys are four times more likely to be identified with ASD than girls (2). In metropolitan Atlanta, Georgia, which consists of five counties, including Clayton, Cobb, DeKalb, Fulton, and Gwinnett, the prevalence of ASD for both white non-Hispanic and black non-Hispanic children increased from 1996 to 2010 (4). However, disparities in prevalence of ASD remain evident between white children (18.1 per 1,000) compared to black children (14 per 1,000) diagnosed with ASD in 2010 (4).

In addition to ASD prevalence disparities, population-based quantitative studies have reported that a range of ASD diagnosis and service disparities are associated with race, ethnicity, and social class (5-9). A quantitative analysis of Medicaid claims of 406 children in Philadelphia found that black children who received specialty mental health services through Medicaid received more time in treatment before obtaining an ASD diagnosis (5) and were 2.6 times less likely than white children to receive a diagnosis on their first specialty care visit (6). One study that examined racial disparities in identification of ASD in metropolitan Atlanta found that black children were less likely to be identified with milder forms of ASD and more likely to receive the most severe diagnosis compared to white children (7). Other studies found that there are ASD disparities associated with age of diagnosis, access to therapeutic services, and even racial representation in special education programs at schools (9-11). Disparities in early evaluation and ASD diagnosis can significantly affect children with ASD and their families mainly because they delay access to early intervention, which is essential for improved developmental outcomes (11). It is recommended that children with ASD receive twenty or more hours per week of behavioral intervention such as Applied Behavioral Analysis (ABA) therapy (12). However, several studies have found that children with ASD who are from racial and ethnic minority populations and communities are less likely than white children with ASD to access publicly funded community-based services, including early intervention and ABA therapy, and those who do are less likely to receive the recommended intensity of twenty hours per week (12).

Although population-based quantitative studies offer important knowledge of factors associated with delays and/or barriers related to ASD diagnosis and services, this literature is relatively descriptive in nature and does not typically consider interrelated social or structural factors that place children and their families at risk of delayed assessment, diagnosis, and/or services (13). Further, quantitative studies on ASD disparities have little to say about the complex and multi-level challenges faced by caregivers in accessing services for their children after a diagnosis has been made. Knowledge gained from qualitative research offers a more nuanced and contextualized understanding of health disparities based on individual lived experiences situated within the context of social and structural dynamics through which health disparities arise and are sustained, reproduced, and perpetuated (13).

In contrast to quantitative ASD research, there is limited qualitative research based on the experiences of families living in low-income, minority, and underserved communities. A recent review conducted by the second author (JS) found that existing qualitative research on ASD disparities focused on the high cost of ASD services, and lack of competence and training in ASD diagnosis and interventions among healthcare and educational professionals (13). The same study found limited qualitative research that examined structural inequities related to operations of systems of care and the regulatory and policy climate (13). Research on the impacts of caring for a child with ASD in alternative family structures is also limited as well as the responsibility taken on by women in general, who are typically the primary caretakers of children, especially children with disabilities (13-14). Further, the representation of female caregivers of children with ASD in the United States is often uneven, with most voices in qualitative research and mainstream culture being those of married, white, upper-class mothers who have the time, social capital, and financial resources to seek early diagnosis and acquire expertise and knowledge on how to help their children (13-15). Our research was informed by these gaps in the existing literature on ASD disparities.

The purpose of this study was to investigate and identify structural inequities that are embedded in the process of navigating state Medicaid insurance for ASD services in Georgia. We define structural inequities as customs, practices, or laws that shape health disparities, including healthcare policies and state programs. Medicaid is a federal program that helps with medical costs for low-income individuals, but how it is designed, managed, and implemented differs from state-to-state (16). There is a long history of the positive impact of Medicaid policy on statewide access to care for low-income and minority adults and children (17). For example, reliance on

Medicaid has been found to be associated with less out-of-pocket medical expenses and reduced financial burden on families (17). However, an unequal distribution of Medicaid services exists across the United States (e.g., differences in Medicaid reimbursements for each state) and even within individual states (e.g., differences in county-level spending on education versus healthcare resources) (17-18). Health insurance, including Medicaid, is one factor among many that has an impact on access to services and health outcomes. Thus, we focused on the compounding factors associated with accessing Medicaid ASD services for single black women who rely on state Medicaid insurance. More specifically, this study investigated the constraints of Medicaid that make it difficult for caregivers to access ASD services after children receive an ASD diagnosis.

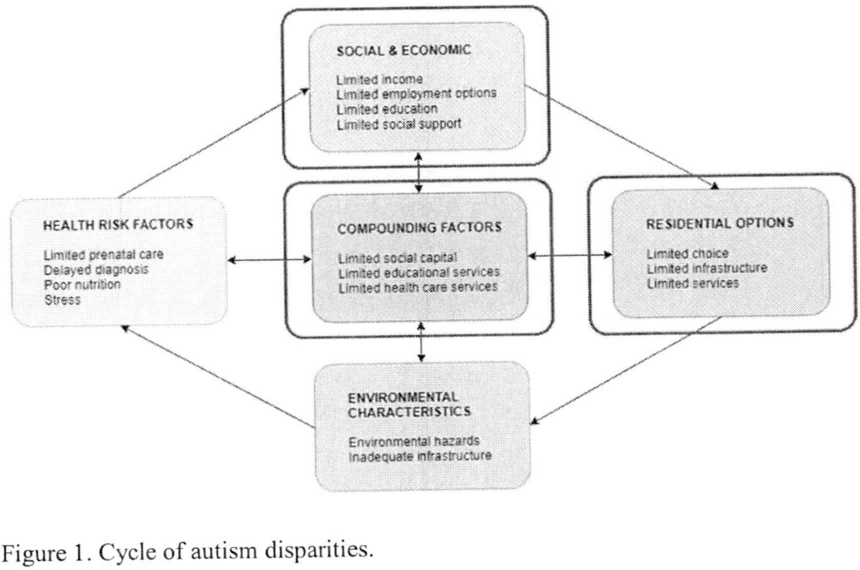

Figure 1. Cycle of autism disparities.

Conceptually, this paper draws on a model (see Figure 1) adapted from the "Cycle of Environmental Health Disparities framework" that outlines the complex environmental interactions in health disparities by identifying a range of interrelated adverse environmental risk factors at the individual, residential, and community levels (19). The "Cycle of Autism Disparities" (see Figure 1) centers on compounding factors (e.g., limited social capital and limited educational and healthcare services) since these factors are central to understanding ASD disparities among underserved communities. For our analysis, we focused on relationships between compounding factors, social and economic factors (e.g., limited education, empowerment, and income), and residential options (e.g., limited choice, infrastructure, and services) portions of the cycle (circled in Figure 1). This model also offered entry points to further expand our understanding of different risk factors associated with ASD service barriers and areas for targeted recommendations to break the cycle of ASD service disparities, which we elaborate in the discussion.

OUR STUDY

This research was approved by Children's Healthcare of Atlanta, Georgia Institute of Technology, and Morehouse School of Medicine Institutional Review Boards, as well as the Grady Research Oversight Committee. Audio-recorded, in-depth interviews were conducted by the second author (JS) with single black female caregivers of children with ASD who rely on state Medicaid health insurance (N = 21). These interviews formed the basis of our analysis and were a subset sample of a larger project designed to assess the quality of care of a community-based Autism Clinic and identify barriers to ASD diagnosis and services (N = 72). Interviews were conducted with caregivers whose children received services at the Autism Clinic located in a non-profit children's hospital in Atlanta, Georgia, where most of the patients rely on Medicaid. Participants were asked open-ended questions about their experiences before, during, and after receiving a diagnosis. All interviews were recorded, transcribed, and uploaded in HyperRESEARCH, a qualitative data analysis software program (20). All the participants were given a pseudonym in the presentation of our findings to protect their confidentiality.

This study used a grounded theory analysis of the interviews to systematically identify themes and multi-level barriers to ASD services (21). This involved using HyperRESEARCH to code segments of qualitative data to specific categories and write detailed memos for categories to capture the data conceptually. Analysis began with open coding of words, phrases, and passages in the interview transcripts. Open coding is an established analytic method used in studies guided by grounded theory methodology, whereby participants' responses are compared, and conceptual labels are defined in an iterative process (21). The second author (JS) developed a preliminary codebook, which was refined as we inspected the data multiple times. The codebook was used to identify common themes shared by participants that reflected and further elaborated the Cycle of Autism Disparities framework (see Figure 1).

FINDINGS

The ability of single black female caregivers to access early intervention and appropriate services through Medicaid insurance after receiving an ASD diagnosis were often compromised due to multiple interacting factors apparent in the Cycle of Autism Disparities framework. Of the sample interviewed, all the study participants identified as black or African American, were single, either never married or divorced, and their children relied on state Medicaid insurance (see Table 1). Sixteen of the caregivers were mothers, and five were grandmothers. Fifty-seven percent of the caregivers were unemployed, thirty-eight percent did not have a college degree, eighty-five percent had a household income of less than $30,000 a year. (Note: the federal poverty level for a four-person household in 2018 was $25,100 (22)). Previous studies on ASD disparities have shown that lower income and/or parental education are associated with lower ASD prevalence, later diagnosis, and less utilization of ASD-related services (12) Thus, the demographics alone place these women at higher risk of experiencing disparities in ASD services. Forty-three percent of the women in the sample also resided in the southern part of Fulton County, an area marked by limited healthcare resources, limited services in public schools, and lower median household income (23). Relatedly, sixty-seven percent of the women in this sample rented an apartment or home or were living in temporary housing (e.g., shelters), and twenty-nine percent took care of more than one child diagnosed with ASD. As we will elaborate below, the interaction of these demographic characteristics is evident in the Cycle of Autism Disparities (see Figure 1), including how limited healthcare resources and educational services (Compounding Factors) available in southern Fulton County (Residential Options) interact with caregivers' educational attainment, income, and employment status (Social and Economic) and their ability to coordinate and access services for their children.

Table 1. Participant demographics (N = 21)

Demographic	**Percent of Sample**
African American or black	100%
Single Parent or Divorced	100%
Medicaid	100%
Unemployed	57%
Some High School/Diploma/Vocation	62%
Household Income <20K	52%
Household Income 20K – 30K	33%
Live in south Fulton County	43%
Rent Apartment / House or Temporary Housing	67%
More than one child diagnosed with ASD	29%

A unique feature about this sample was the fact that these families had access to initial evaluation and diagnosis, which was covered through Medicaid. Most of these families received initial evaluation and diagnosis at the Autism Clinic (69%), while others received initial diagnosis elsewhere (31%). Although access to early evaluation and diagnosis was not the focus of this analysis, caregivers in our sample expressed that "not knowing much about autism," complicated schedule coordination, and long waiting lists were the predominant barriers to early diagnosis. Despite improvements over the last few decades in diagnosing children from racial and ethnic minority communities with ASD in Atlanta, the women in this study continued to experience significant barriers when it came to accessing ASD services such as behavioral, speech, or occupational therapy (2). Thus, their stories reveal how Medicaid served as an access point to obtain an ASD evaluation, diagnosis, and service referrals, while at the same time Medicaid served as a barrier in accessing subsequent ASD services especially in certain geographical locations in metro Atlanta. Two themes were identified that contextualize Medicaid as a barrier to ASD services: bureaucratic processes and geographic location of services.

Bureaucratic processes

It was clear from the stories told by these mothers and grandmothers (24% of sample) that difficulties in accessing services for their children can be contextualized by the complex and often confusing bureaucracy of acquiring ASD services in Georgia. Many caregivers in our sample voiced their confusion and frustration regarding how Medicaid did not cover some of the recommended services for their children or only covered services for a short period of time. Navigating bureaucratic systems is even more difficult because requests for services are lengthy to process, which can result in delays or long waits for caregivers to acquire the appropriate services for their children. Chantel, the mother of a ten-year-old child diagnosed with ASD and another nine-year-old child who displayed developmental delays and behavioral issues, was no stranger to lengthy wait times and limited services available through Medicaid. After being referred to the Autism Clinic for an initial ASD evaluation, it took almost a year for her to secure an appointment for her older child. It was at this first appointment that this child received a diagnosis of ASD. As part of his recommended treatment, Chantel's ten-year-old child did occupational therapy at a rehabilitation center for three months. Although she found occupational therapy helpful for her child in improving his fine motor skills, she ultimately had to discontinue the therapy after Medicaid stopped covering it after three months. At the time of the interview, Chantel had also been looking for a speech therapist for over a year that accepted Medicaid near her home in south Fulton County. Traveling far distances was not a practical option either because Chantel also had to take care of her younger, nine-year-old child who was scheduled to be evaluated for ASD. Chantel was further discouraged by her inability to follow up on referrals received at subsequent appointments for her ten-year-old son because those referrals "did not take Medicaid."

Another young single mother from south Fulton County named Tianna echoed Chantel's sentiments and had difficulties finding an occupational therapist who would accept Medicaid for her five-year-old son diagnosed with ASD. Tianna was the mother of four children and worked full-time as a janitor. Tianna was frustrated because the Medicaid referrals she received from the Autism Clinic were booked and did not have a wait list. As she explained,

> "When I called to schedule an appointment, they said they were booked. There was no waiting list, and they didn't have anyone who could see him because I wanted later hours."

Even though there are other private therapy options available outside Medicaid—which were often located farther away in the northern part of metro Atlanta—Chantel and Tianna could not afford them, and even if they could afford the out-of-pocket cost of these services, they would have to sacrifice their work hours or attention given to their other children. These examples illustrate how limited health care services (Compounding Factors), single parenthood and limited income (Social and Economic), and location of residence (Residential Options) interact with one another in the Cycle of Autism Disparities.

The bureaucratic limitations of Medicaid are compounded when additional institutions are involved. Children with ASD have needs that straddle both healthcare and educational systems. Special educational services for children with ASD are mandated under the Individuals with Disabilities Education Act (IDEA), a federal law that requires a free and appropriate public education be available to children with disabilities in defined age ranges (24). An Individualized Education Program (IEP), which includes a full evaluation of the child with regards to development, speech, or attention, is required for most children to be eligible for services under

IDEA in order to receive special education services in public schools (24). Several caregivers in this study discussed their frustrations with the bureaucratic process required to receive or change an IEP. Sasha, for example, was the mother of a teenaged daughter diagnosed with ASD. Sasha and her three children relocated to Atlanta from North Carolina and at the time of the interview, she was unemployed, financially dependent on her oldest child's income, and lived in a shelter in south Fulton County. Although Sasha first became concerned with her daughter's development when she was an infant, her daughter did not receive a diagnosis of ASD until she was in the sixth grade (when she was around ten years old), at which time Sasha tried to change her daughter's IEP. Due to the time it took to process the necessary paperwork to amend the IEP, Sasha was not able to get her daughter in the "right class" until she started the seventh grade:

> "I had to wait until she graduated sixth grade even though she had a diagnosis of autism."

Sasha went on to say how difficult it was to change her daughter's IEP from a "behavioral intervention class to an autism class," which Sasha believed was more appropriate because the class focused on autism and therefore potentially more beneficial for her daughter.

Another caregiver pointed out an additional complication regarding bureaucratic processes: the educational and medical systems often did not align when it came to evaluations. This caregiver was the mother of six children, and three of her children were diagnosed with ASD. As this mother elaborated,

> "Yeah, [the school] bases [the IEP] on their school system evaluation and not the medical records. Not the doctor's notes. Nothing dealing with your doctor. You may have a child that has autism or other behavior issues that needs to be in a smaller-setting classroom, but when [the school] tests them, and it's not to their liking…Dealing with the school system is like dealing with a whole another government. They have their own set of rules, and personally, you know, for me, I think it's hurting the child to be honest."

These narratives highlight the complicated bureaucratic processes embedded with both the medical and educational public systems and how navigation of these processes for single women with limited resources shape disparities to ASD services.

Geographic location of services

Another salient and recurring theme is how geographic location of services was identified as a constraint to obtaining ASD services. For example, let us consider the experiences of Cynthia, a parent of three children diagnosed with ASD. She resided in south Fulton County, the father of the children was not involved, and she had limited social support from other family members. Alongside the bureaucratic frustrations that came with trying to secure healthcare for her children, Cynthia was frustrated about the limitations of Medicaid coverage and the lack of services around where she lived. Cynthia felt her options were limited because her children were reliant on Medicaid and noted that "there are not many doctors, medical professionals that take the Medicaid." When asked about her biggest challenges in accessing behavioral therapy for her children, Cynthia answered:

> "Well, I can say the area I live… [and] the locations of some of the places that offer the services are…not in my local area, so I have to drive a great distance to get the services. So that's the biggest challenge. There's nothing in my area within a twenty-mile radius, so I have to drive to get there."

Cynthia fortunately had access to the use of a car, which helped her reach therapies that were more than twenty miles away. However, for many of the women in this study, transportation served as a challenge because they relied on public transportation or Medicaid transportation, both of which were not always reliable or practical given these women's demanding life schedules. Caregivers who utilized Medicaid transportation noted that the van was often time-consuming and unreliable. One mother described an incident where she had to reschedule an appointment for her daughter because the Medicaid van was delayed in picking them up. Another mother noted how she found herself late to several appointments at the Autism Clinic because the van often serviced multiple people:

> "You're not the only one riding that van. They have other clients, other customers they have to pick up, as well as pick you up and drop you off. So, you have to sometimes wait until they pick up those guys, and you might be the second or third or fourth person being dropped off…And sometimes, you might be the last person to get dropped off."

In addition, the services these women needed to access for their children were often not easily accessible by public transportation. One grandmother, Karen, who resided in south Fulton County expressed how she was unable to take her three-year-old grandchild diagnosed with ASD to an afterschool learning center that provided services to help children with developmental disabilities:

> "A lot of places are too far. We have no way of getting there. Because of transportation issues…Some of the places are just too far and off the bus line, and I don't have a vehicle, so it makes it harder for me, you know."

At the time of the interview, Karen was recovering from a stroke which she attributed to stress experienced from raising her grandchildren in addition to her own eleven-year-old daughter. Karen was also in the process of adopting her three-year-old grandchild (as well as two other grandchildren who were not diagnosed with ASD). Karen's frustration with transportation issues was felt by parents who owned or had access to a car, but it was heightened for those who had to rely on public transportation.

To add insight into the structural inequities in ASD services in metro Atlanta, a representation of how ASD services are unequally distributed based on geographical location is depicted in Figure 2. The map shows a sample of the places that offer behavioral therapy for ASD. As the map illustrates, there is a lack of behavioral therapy service sites in southern

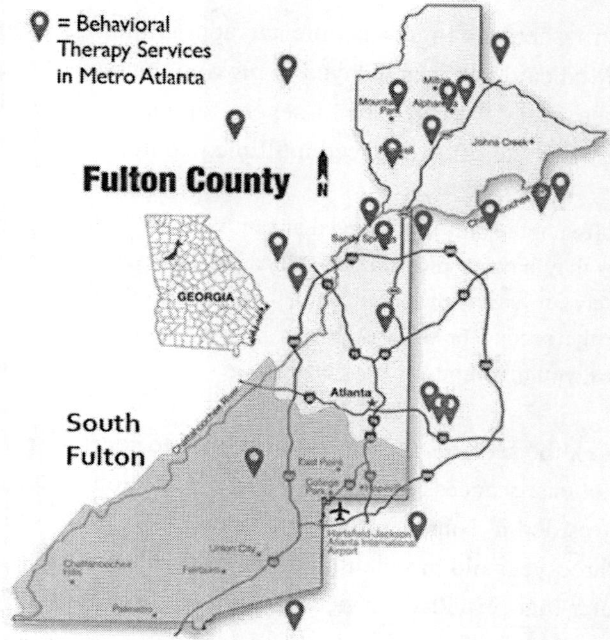

Figure 2. Behavioral therapy services in and around Fulton County.

Atlanta, such as south Fulton County (shaded in darker grey area at the bottom in Figure 2) where Cynthia and forty-three percent of the women in this study live. Those sites that offer behavioral therapy were also often difficult to access with public transportation, and not all of the sites represented in Figure 2 accept state Medicaid insurance. The lengthy travel time to therapies further compound the recommended hours of behavioral therapy per week, which is recommended at more than twenty hours per week (12). In addition, managing work and family life balance for caregivers could be especially challenging if children receive multiple therapies and/or have other healthcare needs in addition to ASD or if parents take care of more than one child with ASD (six parents in our sample had more than one child diagnosed with ASD).

Compounding factors

The challenges associated with both the complex bureaucracy and limited location of services are compounded with other factors evident in Cycle of Autism Disparities framework (see Figure 1). First, these women's challenges were complicated by limited employment options, low income, and stressful environments they and their families must navigate on a daily basis. For example, having to rely on public transportation with a child diagnosed with ASD compounds the challenges these women experience while navigating ASD services. Some of the women told stories of how public transportation created environments that were often difficult for their children to handle due to strange smells, loud noises, large crowds, and long wait times. Sheila, a single black mother who just moved to Atlanta with her teenaged daughters, reflected on how she and her fifteen-year-old daughter diagnosed with ASD could not reach their appointments because her daughter refused to take public transportation,

> "Sometimes I was having trouble with her getting on the train and on the bus…Sometimes she doesn't want to ride. Since the doctor has been helping with the medicine, it's not as bad as before. Before, I couldn't even take her on the bus when there was a whole bunch of people. Because she would have episodes, or she thought people were staring at her."

Also complicating access to care were the barriers related to the consequences of being a single parent, which for this sample was related to navigating ASD services with limited resources and reliance on state services like those supported by Medicaid. Sasha, the previously mentioned mother who encountered problems changing her daughter's IEP, described the difficulties of being a single parent who cares for a child with ASD alongside the multiple responsibilities she faces:

> "If you have a child that has a disability it's even more pressure on me because it's like I have to be Superwoman for everybody else. I still have to deal with regular stuff and on top of regular stuff, deal with other stuff. Sometimes it's kind of overwhelming when you don't have that partner

there to help you…I have to go every place to take to her therapist appointment, her speech appointment. I have to go to her school for IEPs, you know. I have to do a lot…My other daughter who's younger than her, she still has stuff I have to do with her for her school…Then my oldest daughter, even though she's twenty-seven, I still have to be her momma to her too because she has things that's going on in her job."

Additionally, in many cases parents of children with ASD may find their ability to work during their designated employed work hours periodically constrained, which can be especially challenging for single parents (25). For example, Janice, a full-time nursing assistant and the mother of a four-year-old child diagnosed with ASD, was asked to leave her previous job due to the demands of taking care of a child and the toll it took on her work life:

"I made a lot of sacrifices. My other job, I really loved my other job, but I had to leave it due to me leaving work early. Like, if [my child] has a big meltdown, nobody could control him, so I had to leave work and go see him. My supervisor sat me down, and she was like, "You've been taking a lot of days off." I told her what was going on, but she said, "You can stay, or you can leave." I had to leave because this is my son, and I left that company. You know, I really loved that company, but I'm the care provider, I'm his mom, I'm his only parent, and I don't want to ever feel like I'm neglecting him because I'm trying to go to work."

This compelling statement highlights the negotiations that single working women have to contemplate to meet the needs of their child with ASD and the limits on what they can do in their jobs and lives. This caregiver, like many others, must balance the needs of her child with a desirable job, not to mention a job that she needs to support her son. Unfortunately, Janice's employer did not offer the flexibility she needed to manage being the primary breadwinner *and* the primary caregiver. These are conflicts single female caregivers must face, which is compounded when caring for a child with special healthcare needs.

Though this paper focused on the shortcomings of autism services offered through public medical and educational systems, several of the women interviewed were able to quickly acquire services for their children with little difficulty. These women often had financial and/or social support from the fathers of their children or other family members. Some women had the education and knowledge resources to navigate different and equally complex bureaucratic systems. For example, Janice had a bachelor's degree and due to her job as a nursing assistant, had extensive knowledge about Medicaid services and how to acquire various therapies for her son. Janice also sought help and information from a coordinator at the Autism Clinic to arrange multiple therapies for her son. Unlike many of the women in our sample, Janice was able to have her child access several different types of therapies and activities through Medicaid, including speech therapy occupational therapy, physical therapy, swimming lessons, and soccer. These alternative experiences within the sample highlights the heterogeneity of the population under investigation and the importance of having different forms of empowerment and social capital among caregivers in order to navigate complex bureaucratic systems of care. Though public medical and educational programs have enhanced and improved the ability of disadvantaged populations to receive healthcare and related services, ultimately there continues to be areas for improvement.

Discussion

These narratives of single black women negotiating ASD services in metropolitan Atlanta offer firsthand accounts of frustrations that caregivers encounter in dealing with multiple bureaucratic systems of care. These results are in line with a body of research that suggests that when multiple systems are responsible for providing related services to the same child, it can result in considerable gaps and inefficiencies in care (18). The fragmented systems of care and the amount of work required to gain access to state programs and special education services are constraints that are compounded for low-income single, black, female caregivers who are typically doing all the care coordination with limited assistance and/or resources. One avenue to break the cycle of ASD disparities is to consider how medical and educational state programs can work together in offering complementary services for complex conditions like ASD. For example, some researchers have made the case that social workers and occupational therapists who have contact with families of young children might support in early identification and appropriate referrals (26-27). Another study found that increased school district funding was correlated with higher proportions of children identified with ASD in schools (28). Because schools play an important role in identifying children with ASD and other developmental disorders, allocating financial resources and personnel trained to identify ASD to schools in economically disadvantaged communities may help alleviate ASD disparities (28).

Expanding the location of ASD services also points to areas where we can break the cycle of ASD disparities. The experiences of these families who live in south Fulton County highlight how Residential Options (e.g., limited healthcare services in geographic area) and a range of Social and Economic Factors as indicated above. These interrelated factors also matter with regards to race and social class. For example, according to data generated by the US Census, the racial demographics and median household income in Fulton County are starkly different for north Fulton and south Fulton County. For example, in the East Point subdivision of south Fulton County, Blacks account for 79.1 percent of the population, and the median household income was $35,974 in 2010 (23). By contrast in the Roswell-Alpharetta subdivision of north Fulton County, blacks made up only 12 percent of the population (whites composed 61.6 percent of the population here), and the median household income was $97,291 in 2010 (23). We know that higher socioeconomic status (SES) correlates with higher ASD prevalence estimates (29). However, less is known about the effects of compounding factors like living in a lower SES neighborhood that is racially divided. Our data suggests that these are important areas for further investigation. Previous research by Mandell et al. (18) have found that differences in local policies, practices, and resources could result in variation in which children with ASD receive care in the Medicaid system. In our study, difficulties in accessing services can be further contextualized by the lack of services around where these women live and lack of access to reliable transportation if services are farther away. Thus, in addition to addressing the limited ASD services available in low-income and underserved communities, such services should also be made available close to public transportation lines and/or offer transportation services as part of the therapy. The creation of therapy clinics that offer multiple ASD services in one place may also eliminate the constraints placed on caregivers who must travel to multiple locations to acquire different therapies for their children.

As evident by these narratives, the intersecting constraints of trying to access ASD services as a single parent with limited resources highlight how various elements of the Cycle of Autism Disparities framework interact with one another. Several scholars have written about how the accumulation of demands has more consequential effects on populations who have fewer resources to manage their children's ASD (13). For the women in this study, the knowledge, time, and energy necessary to navigate ASD services were compounded by the various challenges related to being a single parent. For example, single parents carry the burden of both unwaged and waged labor (30-31). In this case the unwaged labor consists of navigating the bureaucratic processes needed to obtain ASD services in addition all the other caregiving work required to raise a child with special needs. Previous research also found that achieving and maintaining employment was more difficult for parents of children with disabilities than for those without children or without children with disabilities (25, 32). Cidav et al. (32) found that mothers of children with ASD earn fifty-six percent ($14,755) less than mothers of children with no health limitations, and they are less likely to be employed and work seven hours less per week, on average, than mothers of children with no health limitations. Given the substantial healthcare expenses associated with ASD, the economic impact of having lower income in addition to these expenses is magnified for caregivers of children with ASD (32).

The intersections of gender and race also matter when considering ASD disparities, especially with regards to income inequalities. For example, various studies have shown there are economic sources of inequity due to persistent gender and race differences with regards to types of work that women do and the income they receive (33-34). It was found that irrespective of the level of qualification, jobs predominantly done by women pay less on average than jobs predominantly done by men (33). According to a Pew Research Center analysis of median hourly earnings of both full- and part-time workers in the United States, women earned eighty-three percent of what men earned in 2015 (34). This same study also found that the hourly earnings of black and Hispanic women ($13 and $12, respectively) are lower than those of Asian and white women ($18 and $17, respectively) (34). Our analysis highlights how the challenges of raising a child with ASD was magnified by having limited income, employment options, and social capital (access to knowledge and resources based on one's position in society). These multiple and interrelated factors compounded the difficulties these women experienced in accessing ASD services for their children. While Medicaid coverage lowers financial barriers to accessing healthcare services for low-income uninsured people and improves their health outcomes, the stories these women tell highlight that the program can be further strengthened by addressing recognized shortcomings.

Avenues to break the cycle of ASD disparities must consider these complex and intersecting factors when considering areas of intervention. For example, the development of patient navigation systems designed to provide lay case management especially for families with limited resources early on in ASD evaluation, diagnosis, and services can increase parent empowerment (35). Such programs can be specifically tailored to address issues more apparent for single parent families, such as lack of social support, time, and job flexibility. ASD service disparities among black communities may also benefit from adaption of culturally tailored ASD interventions like the *promotora de salud* model, or community health worker model, to break the cycle for these communities (36). The *promotera de salud* model uses a lay health educator from the target community who provides health information to other people in the target community after receiving training in the health topic (36). For the caregivers of children with ASD in our sample, those with experiences of being single, black, female, and reliant on Medicaid would be the most qualified people to recognize areas of need and areas of strength. For example, a pilot study of parent training for Latinx mothers of children with ASD based on the *promotera de salud* model found that mothers reported improvements in their understanding of ASD, their child's strengths and needs, and how to help their child develop and learn, and knowledge of their child's rights (36). In addition, the study reported that mothers felt improvements in having support systems, accessing the community and using evidence-based approaches efficiently to enhance social communication skills and manage behaviors for children with ASD (36). These suggestions and others can be integrated in community-based settings like preschool and elementary school settings (37-38). Our study supports that it is important to address not only system-level approaches but also the heterogeneity of barriers experienced by under-resourced caregivers of children with ASD (39) Building social capital through such interventions offers important access points to knowledge, resources, and confidence that parents need to break the cycle of ASD service disparities.

CONCLUSION

The examination of ASD disparities in metro Atlanta provides a lens to a bigger problem regarding lack of services in urban areas that are divided based on racial and social class lines. However, the complex bureaucratic processes, lack of services based on geographic location, and interacting compounding factors are also not unique to ASD. People with other disabilities, chronic health problems, and anyone who relies on Medicaid or other state services often face similar challenges. This research focused on the experiences of single black women, whose ability to seek early intervention and appropriate ASD services were often compromised due to multiple compounding factors in a structurally uneven society. The firsthand accounts of the women in this study point to how different processes (Compounding, Social and Economic, and Residential Options) overlap and are contingent on each other. For example, limited health care services are tied to where people live and the choices available for seeking and accessing services. These women's narratives also add more nuance to the Cycle of

Autism Disparities such as the effects of family structure (single parenthood, multiple children with special healthcare needs), the ability to balance work/family life (job flexibility), and transportation options (time, cost, practical considerations)—nuance that opens up and identifies new areas of research and intervention on how to break the cycle of ASD service disparities.

Recent and upcoming changes to Medicaid in the state of Georgia provide avenues for further research as well. In July 2017, the state of Georgia approved a mandate that made it a requirement for Medicaid to cover Adaptive Behavioral Services (ABS) to assess and treat ASD (40). ABS include behavioral therapy and social skills development, and this policy was designed to improve outcomes for ASD. Because nearly half of the women in the sample for this study were interviewed before this mandate was put into effect, the impacts of this mandate currently remain unknown. One research avenue should investigate whether this mandate improves access to ABS and/or increases (or decreases) the bureaucratic processes needed to access these types of ASD services. Further, would such a mandate increase the number of behavioral services in underserved urban areas? The expansion of Medicaid in Georgia through the Patient Protection and Affordable Care Act also holds potential for recipients of Medicaid (41). However, since minorities and women are disproportionately more likely to utilize social assistance programs like Medicaid, these programs are politically vulnerable. As such, recipients are particularly likely to be affected by budget cuts and shoulder the various hardships that accompany reliance on such programs (30-31). Recently in 2019 the Georgia Legislature approved a plan to expand Medicaid, albeit on a limited basis (42-43). There is value in studying the ramifications of Medicaid expansion on healthcare outcomes for low-income, minority, and underserved communities in Georgia. It remains unknown if the limited expansion Medicaid would address the concerns voiced by the women in this study. There is much value in taking note of how recent and upcoming changes to Medicaid in the state of Georgia would affect ASD disparities.

At the individual level, we also have much to learn from the personal stories of the female caregivers themselves, as they provided recommendations to address some of the daily challenges they faced and practical ideas on how to break the cycle of ASD disparities. One recommendation from a mother who worked full-time and could not find an occupational therapist close to her home that accepted Medicaid suggested the integration of Mobile Therapy Units that accept Medicaid in areas like south Fulton County. Such easily transportable therapy services would address the problems related to geographic location of services, as well as create options for offering services in the evenings and/or weekends, when working parents are more likely to be available. One parent voiced her concern that community support groups tended to meet up in Gwinnett or north Fulton County, which are more than twenty miles away and not easily accessible by public transportation. Her suggestion was to create community support groups in south Atlanta that were close to public transportation Southside Support, a community support group based in south Atlanta, was started recently in response to this need (44).

Offering childcare during these sessions (as well as initial therapy sessions) would also allow parents the opportunity to fully engage in these important social support networks. These practical suggestions offer important starting points in breaking the cycle of ASD disparities that may help to alleviate the daunting and often overwhelming task of navigating ASD services among single black women in this study, as well as other families and communities who are situated in similar interacting cycles of health disparities.

ACKNOWLEDGMENTS

This work was supported by Break the Cycle of Environmental Health Disparities 14 and the School of History and Sociology at Georgia Institute of Technology. We would also like to express our gratitude to Dr. Leslie Rubin, the Break the Cycle staff and faculty, and all the women in this study who contributed their valuable time and energy to telling their stories about navigating ASD services.

REFERENCES

[1] American Psychological Association AP. Diagnostic and statistical manual of mental disorders: DSM-5. Washington, DC: American Psychiatric Association, 2013.

[2] Baio J, Wiggins L, Christensen DL, et al. Prevalence of autism spectrum disorder among children aged 8 years: Autism and developmental disabilities monitoring network, 11 sites, United States, 2014. MMWR Surveillance Summary 2018;67(No. SS-6):1-23.

[3] National Research Council. Educating children with autism. Washington, DC: National Academy Press, 2001.

[4] Van Naarden Braun K, Christensen D, Doernberg N, Schieve L, Rice C, Wiggins L, et al. Trends in the prevalence of autism spectrum disorder, cerebral palsy, hearing loss, intellectual disability, and vision impairment, metropolitan Atlanta, 1991-2020. PloS One 2015;10(4):1-21.

[5] Mandell DS, Listerud J, Levy SE, Pinto-Martin JA. Race differences in the age at diagnosis among Medicaid-eligible children with autism. J Am Acad Child Adolesc Psychiatry 2002;41(12):1447-53.

[6] Mandell DS, Ittenbach RF, Levy SE, Pinto-Martin JA. Disparities in diagnoses received prior to a diagnosis of autism spectrum disorder. J Autism Dev Disord 2007;37(9):1795-1802.

[7] Jarquin VG, Wiggins LD, Schieve LA, Van Naarden Braun K. Racial disparities in community identification of autism spectrum disorders over time; metropolitan Atlanta, Georgia, 2000–2006. J Dev Behav Pediatr 2011;32(3):179-87.

[8] Fountain C, King MD, Bearman PS. Age of diagnosis for autism: individual and community factors across 10 birth cohorts. J Epidemiol Community Health 2011,65(6):503-10.

[9] Liptak GS, Benzoni LB, Mruzek DW, Nolan KW, Thingvoll MA, Wade CM, Fryer GE. Disparities in diagnosis and access to health services for children with autism: Data from the National Survey of Children's Health. J Dev Behav Pediatr 2008;29(3):152-60.

[10] Boswell K, Zablotsky B, Smith C. Predictors of autism enrollment in public school systems. Except Child 2014;81(1):96-106.

[11] Estes A, Munson J, Rogers SJ, Greenson J, Dawson G. Long-term outcomes of early intervention in 6-year-old children with autism spectrum disorder. J Am Acad Child Adolesc Psychiatry 2015;54(7):580-7.

[12] Angell AM, Empey A, Zuckerman KE. A review of diagnosis and service disparities among children with autism from racial and ethnic minority groups in the United States. Int Rev Res Dev Disabil 2018;55:146-80.

[13] Singh J, Bunyak G. Autism disparities: A systematic review and meta-ethnography of qualitative research. Qual Health Res 2019;29(6):796-808.

[14] Singh, J. Multiple autisms: Spectrums of advocacy and genomic science. Minneapolis, MN: University of Minnesota Press, 2016.

[15] Angell AM, Solomon O. 'If I was a different ethnicity, would she treat me the same?' Latino parents' experiences obtaining autism services. Disabil Soc 2017;32(8):1142-64.

[16] Paradise J, Lyons B, Rowland D. Medicaid at 50. Kaiser Family Foundation. URL: https://www.kff.org/medicaid/report/medicaid-at-50/.

[17] Thomas KC, Parish SL, Rose RA, Kilany M. Access to care for children in the context of state Medicaid reimbursement. Matern Child Health J 2012;16:1636-44.

[18] Mandell DS, Morales KH, Xie M, Polsky D, Stahmer A, Marcus SC. County-level variation in the prevalence of Medicaid-enrolled children with autism spectrum disorders. J Autism Dev Disord 2010;40:1241-6.

[19] Rubin IL, Geller RJ, Martinuzzi K, Howett M, Gitterman BA, Wells L, et al. Break the cycle of environmental health disparities: An ecological framework. Int Public Health J 2017;9(2):115-30.

[20] Researchware. Researchware: Qualitative research software for the analysis of qualitative data. URL: http://www.researchware.com/.

[21] Charmaz KC. Constructing grounded theory: A practical guide through qualitative analysis. London: Sage; 2006.

[22] US Department of Health and Human Services. Federal poverty level (FPL). URL: https://www.healthcare.gov/glossary/federal-poverty-level-fpl/.

[23] US Census Bureau. 2012-2016 American community survey. Washington DC: US Government Printing Office, 2016.

[24] US Department of Education. Individuals with disabilities education act. URL: https://sites.ed.gov/idea/.

[25] Baker DL, Drapela LA. Mostly the mother: Concentration of adverse employment effects on mothers of children with autism. Soc Sci J 2010;47:578-92.

[26] Dabanah S, Parish SL, Turner Brown L, Hooper SR. Early screening for autism spectrum disorders: A primer for social work practice. Child Youth Serv Rev 2011;33(2):265-73.

[27] Gibbs VD. Detection and treatment of autism spectrum disorder by occupational therapy practitioners: Addressing racial disparity in diagnosis. Am J Occup Ther 2017;71(3):7103360010p1-7103360010p4. doi: 10.5014/ajot.2017.016303.

[28] Palmer RF, Blanchard S, Jean CR, Mandell DS. School district resources and identification of children with autistic disorder. Am J Public Health 2005;95(1):125-30.

[29] Durkin MS, Maenner MJ, Baio J, Christensen D, Daniels J, Fritzgerald R, et al. Autism spectrum disorder among US children (2002-2010): Socioeonomic, racial, and ethnic disparities. Am J Public Health 2017;107(11):1818-26.

[30] Quadagno J. Race, class and gender in the US welfare state: Nixon's failed family assistance plan. Am Sociol Rev 1990;55(1):11-28.

[31] Meyer MH. Gender, race, and the distribution of social assistance: Medicaid use among the frail elderly. Gend Soc 1994;8(1):8-28.
[32] Cidav Z, Marcus SC, Mandell DS. Implications of childhood autism for parental employment and earnings. Pediatrics 2012;129(4):617-23.
[33] Hegewisch A, Hartmann H. The gender wage gap: 2018 earnings differences by race and ethnicity. Institute for Women's Policy Research.. URL: https://iwpr.org/publications/gender-wage-gap-2018/.
[34] Patten E. Racial, gender rage gaps persist in U.S. despite some progress. Pew Research Center. URL: https://www.pewresearch.org/fact-tank/2016/07/01/racial-gender-wage-gaps-persist-in-u-s-despite-some-progress/.
[35] Feinberg E, Abufhele M, Sandler J, Augustyn M, Cabral H, Chen N, et al. Reducing disparities in timely autism diagnosis through Family Navigation: Results from a randomized pilot trial. Psychiatr Serv 2016;67(8):912-5.
[36] Magaña SM, Lopez K, Machalicek W. Parents taking action: A psycho-educational intervention of Latino parents of children with autism spectrum disorder. Fam Process 2017;56(1):59-74.
[37] Dykstra JR, Boyd BA, Watson LR, Crais ER, Baranek GT. The impact of the Advancing Social-communication and Play (ASAP) intervention on preschoolers with autism spectrum disorder. Autism 2012;16(1):27-44.
[38] Kasari C, Smith T. Interventions in schools for children with autism spectrum disorder: Methods and recommendations. Autism 2013;17(3):254-67.
[39] Parsons S, Kasari C. Schools at the centre of educational research in autism: Possibilities, practices, and promises. Autism 2013;17(3):251-3.
[40] Georgia Medicaid. Autism spectrum disorder. URL: https://medicaid.georgia.gov/autism-spectrum-disorder.
[41] US Department of Health and Human Services. About the Affordable Care Act. URL: https://www.hhs.gov/healthcare/about-the-aca/index.html.
[42] Kanso D. Senate bill 106: Medicaid waivers could reshape Georgia's health care system and state budget. Georgia Budget and Policy Institute. URL: https://gbpi.org/2019/medicaid-waivers-could-reshape-georgias-healthcare/.
[43] Hart A, Bluestein G. Georgia governor signs health care waiver bill into law. The Atlanta Journal Constitution. URL: https://www.ajc.com/news/state--regional-govt--politics/georgia-governor-signs-health-care-waiver-bill-into-law/S19OvcyLsHnP2zJEZCk8JJ/.sHnP2zJEZCk8JJ/.
[44] Southside Support. URL: https://www.southsidesupport.org/.

In: Child Environmental Health Disparities ISBN: 978-1-53617-823-4
Editors: IL Rubin and J Merrick

Chapter 8

ENGAGING PARENTS OF CHILDREN WITH AUTISM SPECTRUM DISORDER TO IDENTIFY RURAL HEALTH DISPARITIES AND FACTORS RELATED TO DELAYED DIAGNOSIS AND TREATMENT

Amy A Blumling[1,*], MS, CPNP-PC,
Susan Brasher[1], PhD, CPNP
and Jennifer Stapel-Wax[2,3], PsyD
[1]Nell Hodgson Woodruff School of Nursing,
Emory University, United States of America
[2]School of Medicine, Emory University, United States of America
[3]Marcus Autism Center, Atlanta, Georgia, United States of America

* Correspondence: Amy A Blumling, Emory University School of Nursing, 1520 Clifton Rd NE, Atlanta, GA 30322, United States. Email: ablumli@emory.edu.

ABSTRACT

Autism spectrum disorder (ASD) is a developmental disability characterized by significant social, communication, and behavioral challenges. Early diagnosis and treatment have shown to improve health outcomes. ASD diagnosis can be achieved by age 2 years, but median age of diagnosis is 4-5 years. The purpose of this project is to identify barriers and facilitators to ASD diagnosis and treatment for families living in rural or Medically Underserved Areas (MUAs). Methods: Two focus groups were conducted online and in-person with parents of children with ASD living in rural and MUAs. Questions examined health disparities and delayed diagnosis or treatment. Sessions were audio-recorded, transcribed, and analyzed. Results: Diagnosis and treatment barriers included distance to healthcare services, limited access to providers, inadequate insurance coverage, and lack of education. Facilitators included school referrals, research studies, ASD research centers, support groups, school-based treatments, and insurance extenders. Analysis revealed decreased parental autonomy, frustration, disappointment, uncertainty, and desire for support. Discussion: Parents of children with ASD living in rural and MUAs discussed several barriers to ASD diagnosis and treatment. Parent-identified ways to improve barriers included increased education, enhanced awareness of ASD and needs of rural and MUAs, and improved access to care. Proposed interventions included telehealth and mobile clinics. Conclusion: Families living in rural and MUAs face many barriers related to ASD diagnosis and treatment. Future interventions should address these issues by increasing awareness of ASD, increasing knowledgeable providers, and utilizing electronic technologies to engage individuals in these areas.

INTRODUCTION

Autism spectrum disorder (ASD) is a complex neurodevelopmental disorder characterized by communication, social, and behavioral challenges for affected individuals (1). ASD is associated with a variety of both personal and family-level challenges, including the need for lifelong support and interventions. Families of children with ASD living in rural or medically underserved areas (MUAs) face additional challenges in obtaining a diagnosis and securing ongoing treatment due to a variety of factors, which results in potential healthcare disparities present in these populations (2-4).

There is currently a scarcity of research on families of children with ASD living in rural and MUAs and the role that disparities in services plays in the diagnosis and treatment of ASD. Therefore, the purpose of this project was to identify barriers and facilitators to ASD diagnosis and treatment for families living in rural or MUAs.

AUTISM SPECTRUM DISORDER

Symptoms of ASD emerge in early childhood and include difficulty with communication, difficulty with social-emotional reciprocity, and the presence of restrictive and repetitive behaviors or interests (1). The current prevalence of ASD is estimated to affect 1 in 59 children (5). In addition to the primary characteristics of ASD, children with ASD encounter numerous health and behavioral comorbidities (e.g., seizures, gastrointestinal disorders, attention-deficit/hyperactivity disorder [ADHD], sleep disorders), increasing the complex needs of these children (5, 6). Treatment for ASD includes evidence-based treatments, such as applied behavioral analysis (ABA) therapy, speech language pathology (SLP), occupational therapy (OT), and physical therapy (PT). As a result of the complex nature of ASD and its associated treatment, the lifetime cost of supporting a single individual with ASD in the United States is estimated to be between $1.4-2.4 million (7). Despite this costly economic burden on individuals and families, evidence has shown that early diagnosis and intervention for children with ASD can improve long-term health outcomes (7-10).

Given that signs and symptoms of ASD appear in the first year of life, clinicians are currently able to make a valid diagnosis as early as two years of age (1). According to emerging literature, this age may actually be sooner for some children with ASD. (5, 8, 9, 11). Despite these facts, the current median age that children receive an ASD diagnosis is between 4-5 years (2, 5, 8-10). This delay in ASD diagnosis delays the child's ability to receive treatment services, resulting in a significant lag between presentation of symptoms and onset of intervention. This delay has great potential to negatively impact the developmental trajectory of the child, as it occurs during a critical time of early brain development (8-11). Evidence has shown that a timely ASD diagnosis, coupled with early intervention, increases the likelihood of favorable long-term health outcomes (8, 9, 11).

Rural and medically underserved areas (MUAs)

Geographic health disparities are associated with individuals living in rural or MUAs, where access to care affects their ability to receive necessary healthcare treatments. The United States Health Resources and Service Administration (HRSA) defines rural areas as those that have fewer than 2,500 people (12). MUAs are defined as areas that have too few primary care providers, high infant mortality, high poverty, and/or a high elderly population (13, 14). While limited access to healthcare services in rural areas may appear evident, often overlooked are those residing in MUAs who face even higher health adversities and disadvantages given their unique disparities. Research has found that individuals who are part of disadvantaged populations (e.g., geographic, socioeconomic, racial, ethnic) experience comparatively poorer outcomes in health (15-17). Thus, delayed diagnosis and treatment of any health-related problem are more detrimental to the health outcomes of these disadvantaged populations (2-4, 17-20).

It is currently estimated that nearly one in five Americans live in rural areas and often struggle to meet their healthcare needs due to a lack of providers (21). As of 2018, there were a total of 4,118 primary care health professional shortage areas identified in rural locations compared to only 1,960 in urban locations, thus increasing the vulnerability of these populations, as they are considered to be both medically underserved and living in a rural area (21). As a result, life expectancy rates can vary by up to 20 years based on an individual's geographic location (16, 22). At present, Georgia ranks in the lowest quartile in terms of life expectancy by state (16, 22), where nearly 90% of Georgia counties are designated as rural or MUAs (see Figure 1).

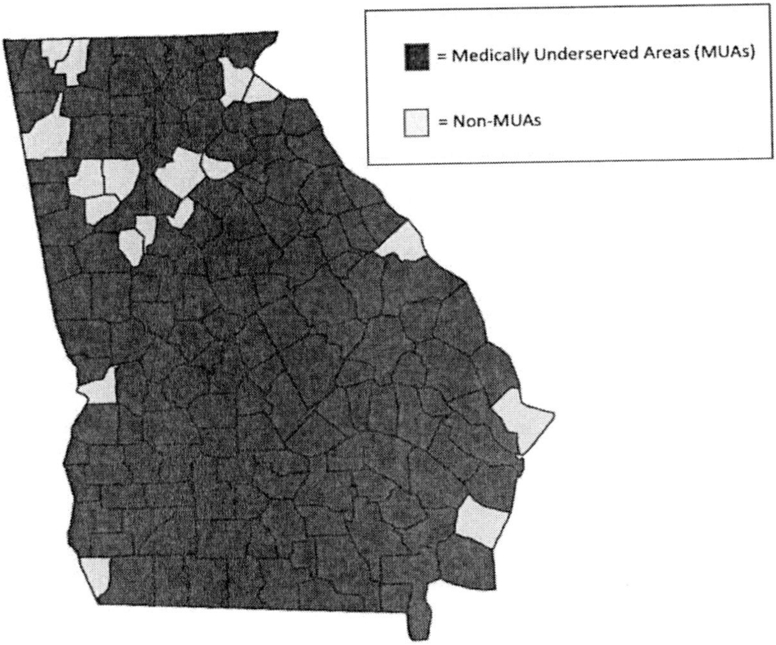

Figure 1. Map of medically underserved areas by county in the State of Georgia.

Cycle of children's health disparities

Health disparities are present in children and families who have limited financial, social, medical, therapeutic, and educational resources. These disparities can be viewed in an intergenerational cycle that includes various geographic, health, environmental, personal, compound risk factors, and environments that can negatively impact a child's health (see Figure 2) (23-28). This project aims to break the cycle of children's health disparities by exploring factors that impact families of children with ASD living in rural or MUAs, as indicated by the asterisks in Figure 2. As a result of this investigation, we intend to propose strategies to improve the health of children and families (see Figure 2).

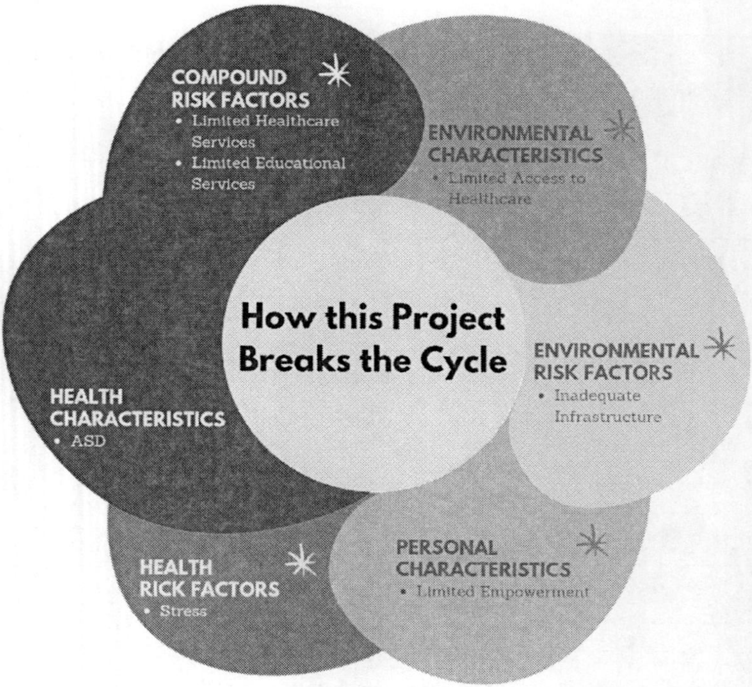

Figure 2. Breaking the cycle of autism health disparities in rural and MUAs.

OUR STUDY

The principal study investigators recruited parents of children with ASD living in rural and MUAs of Georgia to explore barriers and facilitators to ASD diagnosis and treatment. The study was deemed exempt by the Emory University Institutional Review Board (IRB). Recruitment took place through flyers sent to local and rural pediatric clinics, social media support groups, and collaborative partners (e.g., Marcus Autism Center, Emory Autism Center, Department of Education Parent Mentors). Two focus groups were held, one in person and one online using remote, Health Insurance Portability and Accountability Act of 1996 (HIPAA)-compliant video-conferencing technology (i.e., Zoom) (29). The two groups consisted of three to ten participants each, and they included parents of children with

ASD and an additional stakeholder, the director of a special education school.

Focus groups utilized open- and closed-ended questions to identify potential barriers and facilitators to delayed ASD diagnosis and treatment. Questions also explored family-centered solutions to mitigate any potential disparities (see Table 1). The focus groups were audio recorded, transcribed, and analyzed using thematic analysis.

Table 1. Focus group guide

Focus group questions
1. Do you think there are any barriers or facilitators to receiving your child's ASD diagnosis?
2. Tell me more about these barriers or facilitators.
3. Do you think there are any barriers or facilitators to receiving treatment for your child?
4. Tell me more about these barriers or facilitators.
5. What do you think should be done to help families get an earlier diagnosis or treatment?

FINDINGS

Participants represented numerous counties throughout the state of Georgia, some of which were up to 200 miles apart. Because of the interest from counties that were dispersed throughout the state, researchers decided to employ an innovative method for conducting qualitative research: utilizing both in-person and online videoconference focus groups. During the focus groups, participants discussed their perceptions of barriers and facilitators to early ASD diagnosis and treatment.

Geographic diversity

Initial participant recruitment resulted in high interest from a variety of geographically diverse locations throughout the state of Georgia. Interested participants spanned nine different counties dispersed throughout Georgia, including Walton, Troup, Fayette, Liberty, Bulloch, Sumter, Columbia, Henry, and Appling Counties (see Figure 3). The geographic diversity and distance in the sample compelled the researchers to conduct one of the focus groups online. This offered participants in a variety of counties a chance to have their voices heard in this study, despite the fact that their distant geographic location would have normally precluded them from participating in traditional in-person focus groups.

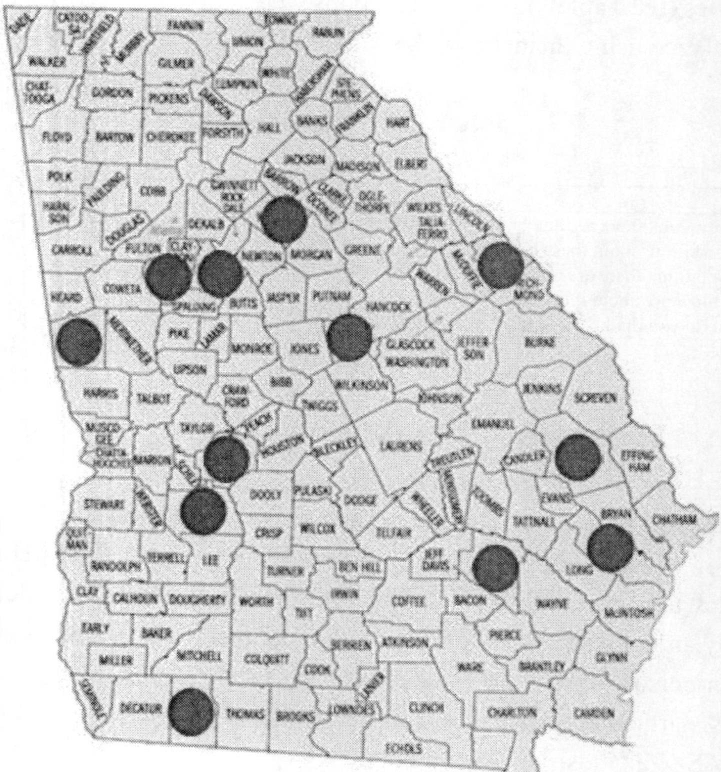

Figure 3. Georgia county map of interested participants.

Diagnosis

Barriers and facilitators to ASD diagnosis were among the most frequently discussed topics during the focus groups. Parents living in rural and MUAs in Georgia felt that their experiences in receiving an ASD diagnosis differed from individuals living in more heavily populated areas, or areas with more providers.

Table 2. List of barriers and facilitators to ASD diagnosis and treatment

	Barriers	Facilitators
Diagnosis	• Distance to health care providers • Provider shortages • Inadequate insurance coverage • Lengthy wait times for providers • Lack of parental and provider education on ASD signs and symptoms • Limited ASD awareness of providers	• School system referrals • Working with ASD research centers • Participating in research studies
Treatment	• Distance to health care providers • Limited providers in immediate area • Inadequate insurance coverage • Cost of treatments • Competing time demands • Lack of follow-up plans for the child	• Social media support groups • Insurance extenders • Access to school-based treatments

Barriers

Parents described their journey to receiving an ASD diagnosis as being filled with various barriers that ultimately created a great burden to their family. The main barriers identified were distance to health care providers, provider shortages, inadequate insurance coverage, lengthy wait times, lack of parental and provider education on ASD, and limited ASD awareness of providers (see Table 2). Parents discussed problems with their initial concerns being dismissed by providers, lengthy wait times to see providers capable of making an ASD diagnosis, and limited providers working in their native counties. They also expressed frustration and disappointment in finding a lack of education and awareness about their child's developmental concerns. Numerous concerns with insurance arose that impeded a child's ability to receive a timely diagnosis, specifically providers capable of making an ASD diagnosis not accepting certain insurance. Limited providers in the area, combined with dissatisfaction with the available providers, led many parents to seek providers outside their immediate counties. This often required them to travel upwards of two hours roundtrip for a single appointment to discuss their child's signs and symptoms.

Quotes from parents related to diagnosis barriers

The following quotes from parents represent the variety of barriers that parents living in rural or MUAs in Southern Georgia face in pursuance of an ASD diagnosis for their child:

> Lack of ASD Awareness – Participant 1: "…They just kept telling me that my kid's lazy, that boys are lazy, and that's what I was being told the whole time."
>
> Limited Providers & Lengthy Wait Times – Participant 2: "…There is nowhere around here that I knew of, or that at the time, my pediatrician knew of… that could give the autism diagnosis other than [large autism centers], [both] of which at the time was on an extremely long waiting list."

Facilitators

Although parent participants heavily emphasized the barriers to early diagnosis, they also discussed some facilitators that helped the process of diagnosis (see Table 2). Facilitators to diagnosis included school system referrals, working with large ASD centers, and participating in research studies. Parents felt that these facilitators improved early diagnoses. Examples of how these processes facilitated an earlier diagnosis included educators having a developmental concern for a child and making a school-based referral, having access to large ASD centers where professionals are specifically trained in ASD diagnosis and treatment, and opportunities for parents to have their child in research studies that provided ASD diagnosis and/or treatment (e.g., studies that evaluate siblings of children with ASD for developmental delays). Additionally, parents mentioned that their own persistence and determination in pursuing a diagnosis for their child were the most influential facilitators.

Quote from parent related to diagnosis facilitators

The following quote from a parent represents the facilitators that aided parents in receiving an ASD diagnosis for their child in rural and MUAs:

> Parental Perseverance – Participant 3: "...Most of the parents here, we're the go-getters, we're the advocates. I had learned at an early, younger year, like, I have to fight, fight, fight and not take 'no' [as an answer]…"

Treatment services

Upon receiving an ASD diagnosis, parents discussed factors that impacted receiving treatment services for their child. Accessing follow-up care after the ASD diagnosis and receiving ongoing treatment were often problematic for parents living in rural and MUAs.

Barriers

When identifying barriers to ASD treatments for their child, parents discussed many of the same problems associated with barriers to diagnosis (see Table 2). These treatment barriers included distance, limited providers, insurance, cost, competing demands, and lack of follow-up. Similar to diagnosis barriers, treatment barriers centered around the lack of providers in the immediate area who were able or willing to provide ongoing treatments to children with ASD. Parents also mentioned that the state-wide early intervention programs were not necessarily helpful, as there appeared to be a severe provider shortage for these programs in their rural and MUAs. Of the limited providers available, parents often mentioned that they once again had problems with providers taking certain types of insurance for the treatments. When insurance was unwilling to cover these expenditures, it caused parents to pay out-of-pocket for often expensive interventions. This led to parents seeking providers outside their native counties who would be willing to treat children with ASD, as well as accept their insurance. This ultimately led to problems with competing demands requiring extended time commitments, such as missed school or work days.

Finally, a large problem identified was the lack of follow-up care for parents once they received an ASD diagnosis for their child. Parents expressed that they were relieved once they received the ASD diagnosis, but then felt unsure as to how they were supposed to follow-up or with whom in their native counties for treatment services. Parents described a lack of coordination and clear direction for parents regarding treatments, services, or facilities to seek out after receiving their child's ASD diagnosis.

Quotes from parents related to treatment barriers

The following quotes from parents represent the barriers to treatment and follow-up care for their child with ASD in rural and MUAs in Georgia:

> Limited Providers – Participant 4: "Two different problems…Getting the diagnosis, but then even when you get the diagnosis, that doesn't solve everything [because] then there's not [any] treatments [in rural areas]."
>
> Distance – Participant 5: "I have to drive an hour east or two hours west to go to an appointment. So, he misses school, and it happens because we live in a rural area."
>
> Lack of Follow-Up – Participant 1: "I thought…I was there getting a diagnosis and you're going to help me fix him. And I remember saying, 'well, what next?'"

Facilitators

Aside from the overwhelming barriers to accessing evidence-based treatments, parents identified certain facilitators that enhanced this process (see Table 2). Social media support groups (e.g., Facebook), insurance extenders and access to school-based treatments were identified as facilitators to ASD treatment. Social media groups allowed them to find both helpful resources and support for their experiences. Parents expressed that these social groups helped with the processes involved in applying for services, such as specific treatments or insurance extenders. The insurance extenders, or medical Deeming Waivers (previously known as the Katie Beckett Waiver) (30), allowed families of children with disabilities to apply for Medicaid coverage services without their family income being taken into consideration. Lastly, school-based therapies or school systems that offered evidence-based therapies were found to be facilitators to treatment Unfortunately, few school systems in Southern Georgia were reported to offer such services.

Quotes from parents related to treatment facilitators

The following quotes from parents demonstrate how social media support groups and insurance extenders facilitated treatment for their children:

> Social Groups & Insurance Extenders – Participant 3: "…[Social media groups] … had people talking about the Katie Beckett and trying to…apply for the Katie Beckett was very overwhelming, frustrating. So, they said, you know, hey, there's a specific group that helps you, that does that, so you can post questions in there, or you can search to see if your question's already been asked. And so that group was very helpful."
>
> Social Groups – Participant 6: "I wouldn't have found out about the ABA (Applied Behavioral Analysis) group, the ABA place that opened up in [local location] if it wasn't for the [social media] group."

Parental suggestions for improvement

In addition to identifying the barriers and facilitators to ASD diagnosis and treatment in rural and MUAs in Georgia, parents were asked what should be done going forward to improve ASD diagnosis and treatment for those living in rural and MUAs. Parental suggestions to improve issues of health disparities when navigating the healthcare system for children with ASD included: increased education for parents and healthcare providers on early signs and symptoms of ASD, enhanced public and healthcare awareness of the disorder, increased training of new ASD diagnosticians or treatment providers, better hand-off from diagnosis to treatment, and better access to care in rural and MUAs. While these are strategies that will be universally helpful and facilitative for all children and families with ASD, these ideas are particularly important for families in rural or MUAs who, by virtue of their distance from resources, must take a more informed and active role in the early development of their children and advocacy for their children's' health.

One of the most significant problems reportedly faced by parents in rural and MUAs to receiving an ASD diagnosis and treatment was the lack of education and awareness about ASD in the community, schools, and healthcare. Specifically, they felt that their concerns over early red flags in their children's development were ignored by certain professionals, leading to delays in diagnosis and treatment. They also discussed how other physiological, psychological, or social disorders of childhood received more public attention and awareness compared to ASD. In order to address these concerns, parents suggested increased education, awareness, and training for professionals interacting with children on a daily basis, such as those working in the education system and pediatric-focused medical fields.

In addition to these potential solutions, parents also described how better transitions from diagnosis to treatment and access to care in their native areas would greatly ease the burden of ASD treatments in rural and MUAs. One participant suggested that after leaving an appointment with a provider who could make the ASD diagnosis, that same provider could also specify next steps and contact information to treatment providers. This parent also suggested a document list of providers in their native areas and the insurances these individuals accepted. Other suggestions for increasing access to care in these underserved areas included the following interventions: telehealth, mobile clinics, encouraging other providers to come to the area, and having healthcare students train in rural and MUAs. To implement these ideas, parents suggested the use of telehealth and mobile clinics. They also proposed that healthcare organizations offer incentives to increase the number of providers willing to work in rural and MUAs, as well as partnering with nearby schools to train students in rural areas.

Quotes from parents related to ideas for improvement

The following quotes from parents identified ways to address ASD disparities in diagnosis and treatment in rural and MUAs:

> Mobile Clinics – Participant 7: "I think it will help if they brought like…mini clinics. Even, you know, something a little closer so we don't always have to drive so far out."
>
> Increasing Providers – Participant 8: "I think that, well, there needs to be more developmental pediatricians and…diagnosticians. So, whether it's a psychiatrist, psychologist… that can make the diagnosis."
>
> Training Providers – Participant 2: "…a lot of the schools like [local University] have really big [therapy programs]. In order for students to get their…ABA clinic hours, [they practice delivering ABA therapy to children with ASD]. That's why parents are able to afford it, because now these are college kids doing it for clinic hours."

Discussion

Timely diagnosis and treatment is crucial for the long-term health outcomes of children with ASD. This process can be impeded by a variety of factors, but the challenges are compounded for individuals living in rural or MUAs. Individuals in these areas face a disproportionate number of unique health disparities and barriers related to acquiring a diagnosis and accessing treatment for ASD, when compared to their urban peers (4, 17, 19).

Focus groups with parents of children with ASD living in rural and MUAs revealed a number of barriers related to both ASD diagnosis and treatment. Parents described a variety of diagnosis and treatment challenges, including limited providers in their area, excessive distance to providers, lengthy wait times for appointments, inadequate insurance coverage, lack of parental and provider education, and overall lack of awareness of ASD diagnoses and treatment in both families and clinicians. In addition, parents also mentioned the lack of follow-up care, leaving them feeling unsure of what the next steps were supposed to be after receiving their child's ASD diagnosis. Thematic analysis of parents' responses revealed perceived limited parental autonomy over their child's healthcare, frustration and disappointment with the healthcare system, and a desire for more support and education. The impact of these disparities and barriers weighs emotionally and financially on parents and families in the form of lost jobs due to time away from work to attend appointments, lost time in school for affected children and siblings, and a general sense of confusion and abandonment by the healthcare system. One parent specifically mentioned that due to the distance and necessary time-off that she had to take from her job, she ended up being fired and becoming unemployed, thus creating the cycle of poverty and perpetuating the cycle of health disparities. These barriers not only affect parents and families, but also could potentially influence the affected child's developmental and social health trajectory if not addressed appropriately.

Many rural and MUA areas are underserved, and families of children with ASD in these populations suffer disproportionately compared to their peers; however, little is known in terms of specific barriers and facilitators to diagnosis and treatment, as well as family-based interventions. This study has demonstrated the needs of underserved children and families with ASD residing in rural and MUAs in Georgia, and it addresses them specifically with a desire to know the barriers and facilitators, to engage the community, and to offer partnership in community-based pragmatic solutions. It has also drawn attention to the difficulties in recruitment and engagement of rural communities. Members of these areas are potentially vulnerable families with past negative experiences with healthcare and research, and they may be hesitant to participate in studies without rapport and understanding being built first. They also face challenges with numerous obligations of running a home and family, which renders them unable to participate in-person in studies. However, there are ways to ensure that the voices of individuals from rural and MUAs are heard and are present in ASD research, despite any challenges that arise from their geographic locations and socioeconomic and cultural circumstances.

The use of online focus groups to engage parents living in rural allows the consideration of the pros and cons of conducting non-traditional (i.e., online) focus group research and service in these areas. Positive aspects of these nontraditional focus groups can include the chance for participants who live in distant areas to share their stories and have their voices heard when they might not be able to participate in person otherwise, enabling them to be more empowered. However, potential problems with online focus groups may involve technical difficulties when conducting them or the possibility of missing out on a more personalized, in-person interaction. Despite these challenges, research and medical care utilizing telehealth, mobile clinics, or online resources could potentially mitigate the geographic health disparities in vulnerable communities dealing with access to care difficulties. These solutions offer viable alternatives to traditional diagnostic and therapeutic services in rural and MUAs.

Future directions

Future directions for this study, and for studying ASD disparities in MUAs, involve continuing to engage more parents, especially those living in rural and MUAs in different areas of the state, and in other states with large rural or MUA populations. Research would also benefit from engaging other stakeholders, including providers, educators, parent mentors, and policymakers, to better understand their perspective and experiences with these healthcare disparities. Finally, future research should focus on interventions to minimize these health disparities in MUAs, potentially through the use of telehealth or mobile clinics. Additional interventions, as suggested by the parents, should involve increasing ASD awareness and education to pediatric providers and individuals who work with children, such as those in the school sector. This would likely help to recognize early signs and symptoms of ASD in children and potentially aid in earlier diagnoses. Finally, statewide early interventions may consider leveraging their existing outreach, increasing visibility through social media or other shared programs, and improving existing programs to increase ASD diagnosis.

Limitations

The scope of this project was a pilot project. Thus, the sample size was limited. However, the experience and frustrations expressed by participants in this study are mirrored with other populations. Additionally, given that this population is understudied in the ASD community, the small sample size works as a pilot project for assessing the feasibility for reaching these groups, whether it be via in-person or online focus groups, as many of the families are unable to travel long distances to meet in person. Despite the small sample size, results of this study are an important first step to conducting future research in rural and MUAs, as well as determining feasibility of tele-focus groups. This will increase the generalizability to different populations, and it could potentially lead to the development of evidence-based interventions.

Conclusion

Parents of children with ASD living in rural and MUAs face health disparities in the forms of barriers to accessing ASD diagnosis and treatment. A majority of barriers are centered around the lack of access to providers and challenges associated with access to care, such as limited providers in the area providing ASD specific services and issues with insurance providers not covering treatments. Potential interventions to address these barriers must be focused on patient- and family-centered care, where patients and families identify their specific needs and possible solutions to address them. According to the parents in this study, decreasing health disparities in MUAs in Georgia may be accomplished through increased education, enhanced awareness, and increasing the number of providers that are available to meet the needs of these underserved, vulnerable populations. Given that there are many states throughout the United States that have rural and MUAs similar to Georgia, this early research is key to developing interventions for many children and families affected by ASD healthcare disparities throughout the country. Such interventions could include innovative methods of delivering care, such as through the use of telehealth and mobile clinics, as well as increasing awareness of ASD for parents, providers, and educators of young children These interventions address the factors of limited access to healthcare and educational services, inadequate infrastructure, and limited parental empowerment and stress, thus helping to break the cycle of ASD health disparities in rural and MUAs.

ACKNOWLEDGMENTS

The authors would like to thank the parents and stakeholders in rural and MUAs of Georgia, the Georgia Department of Education, the Pediatric Environmental Health Specialty Unit, and Break the Cycle of Health Disparities, Inc. Disclosures: The authors have nothing to disclose.

REFERENCES

[1] American Psychiatric Association. Diagnostic and statistical manual of mental disorders, 5 ed. Washington, DC: APA, 2013.

[2] Antezana L, Scarpa A, Valdespino A, Albright J, Richey JA. Rural trends in diagnosis and services for autism spectrum disorder. Front Psychol 2017;8:590.

[3] Hutton AM, Caron SL. Experiences of families with children with autism in rural New England. Focus Autism Other Dev Disabil 2005;20(3):180-9.

[4] Mello MP, Goldman SE, Urbano RC, Hodapp RM. Services for children with autism spectrum disorder: Comparing rural and non-rural communities. Educ Train Autism Dev Disabil 2016;51(4):355-65.

[5] Christensen DL, Braun KVN, Baio J, Bilder D, Charles J, Constantino JN, et al. Prevalence and characteristics of autism spectrum disorder among children aged 8 years—autism and developmental disabilities monitoring network, 11 sites, United States, 2012. MMWR Surveill Summ 2018;65(13):1-23.

[6] Levy SE, Giarelli E, Lee L-C, Schieve LA, Kirby RS, Cunniff C, et al. Autism spectrum disorder and co-occurring developmental, psychiatric, and medical conditions among children in multiple populations of the United States. J Dev Behav Pediatrics 2010;31(4):267-75.

[7] Buescher AV, Cidav Z, Knapp M, Mandell DS. Costs of autism spectrum disorders in the United Kingdom and the United States. JAMA Pediatr 2014;168(8):721-8.

[8] Elder JH, Kreider CM, Brasher SN, Ansell M. Clinical impact of early diagnosis of autism on the prognosis and parent–child relationships. Psychol Resd Behav Manage 2017;10:283.

[9] Elder JH, Brasher S, Alexander B. Identifying the barriers to early diagnosis and treatment in underserved individuals with autism spectrum disorders (ASD) and their families: A qualitative study. Issues Ment Health Nurs 2016;37(6):412-20.

[10] Rotholz DA, Kinsman AM, Lacy KK, Charles J. Improving early identification and intervention for children at risk for autism spectrum disorder. Pediatrics 2017;139(2):e20161061.

[11] Zwaigenbaum L, Bauman ML, Stone WL, Yirmiya N, Estes A, Hansen RL, et al. Early identification of autism spectrum disorder: Recommendations for practice and research. Pediatrics 2015;136(Suppl 1):S10-S40.

[12] Health Resources and Services Administration. Defining rural population 2018. URL: https://www.hrsa.gov/rural-health/about-us/definition/index.html.

[13] Health Resources and Services Administration. Medically underserved areas and populations (MUA/Ps) 2019. URL: https://bhw.hrsa.gov/shortage-designation/muap.

[14] Health Resources and Services Administration. MUA Find 2019. URL: https://data.hrsa.gov/tools/shortage-area/mua-find.

[15] Williams DR. The health of US racial and ethnic populations. J Gerontol Series B Psychol Sci Soc Sciences 2005;60(2):S53-S62.

[16] Dwyer-Lindgren L, Bertozzi-Villa A, Stubbs RW, Morozoff C, Mackenbach JP, van Lenthe FJ, et al. Inequalities in life expectancy among US counties, 1980 to 2014: Temporal trends and key drivers inequalities in life expectancy among US counties. JAMA Intern Med 2017;177(7):1003-11.

[17] Hartley D. Rural health disparities, population health, and rural culture. Am J Public Health 2004;94(10):1675-8.

[18] Mandell DS, Novak MM, Zubritsky CD. Factors associated with age of diagnosis among children with autism spectrum disorders. Pediatrics 2005;116(6):1480.

[19] Eberhardt MS, Pamuk ER. The importance of place of residence: examining health in rural and nonrural areas. Am J Public Health 2004;94(10):1682-6.

[20] National Conference of State Legislatures. Meeting the primary care needs of rural America: Examining the role of non-physician providers 2019. URL: http://www.ncsl.org/research/health/meeting-the-primary-care-needs-of-rural-america.aspx.

[21] National Organization of State Offices of Rural Health. About rural health in America 2018. URL: https://nosorh.org/about-rural-health-in-america/.

[22] Centers for Disease Control and Prevention. Life expectancy 2017. URL: https://www.cdc.gov/nchs/fastats/life-expectancy.htm.

[23] PEHSU: SE Pediatric Environmental Health Specialty Unit: Emory University School of Medicine Department of Pediatrics, 2017. URL: http://www.pediatrics.emory.edu/centers/pehsu/index.html.

[24] Rubin IL, Geller RJ, Martinuzzi K, Gitterman BA, Wells L, BSCE WG, et al. Children's environmental health disparities: The costs and benefits of breaking the cycle. Int J Child Health Hum Dev 2016;9(4):419.

[25] Rubin IL, Geller RJ, Martinuzzi K, Gitterman BA, Wells L, BSCE WG, et al. Break the cycle of environmental health disparities: An ecological framework. Int Public Health J 2017;9(2):115.

[26] Finn S. Environmental health literacy. Cham, Switzerland: Springer, 2019.

[27] Landrigan PJ, Rauh VA, Galvez MP. Environmental justice and the health of children. Mt Sinai J Med 2010;77(2):178-87.

[28] Landrigan PJ. What causes autism? Exploring the environmental contribution. Curr Opin Pediatrics 2010;22(2):219-25.

[29] HIPAA Business Associate Agreement (BAA): Zoom. URL https://support.zoom.us/hc/en-us/articles/207652183-HIPAA-Business-Associate-Agreement-BAA-.

[30] Tax Equity and Fiscal Responsibility Act of 1982, Pub. L. No. 97-248(09/03/1982), 1982.

In: Child Environmental Health Disparities ISBN: 978-1-53617-823-4
Editors: IL Rubin and J Merrick

Chapter 9

EVALUATION OF HEALTH LITERACY IN CHILDHOOD-ONSET SYSTEMIC LUPUS ERYTHEMATOSUS PATIENTS AND ITS EFFECT ON HEALTHCARE UTILIZATION

Catherine Park[1,2,*], MD, Traci Leong[3], PhD, Alexandria Wilkerson[1], Christy Kang[1], Margret Kamel[1], PhD, Kelly Rouster-Stevens[2,4], MD, and Roshan George[1,2], MD

[1]Division of Pediatric Nephrology, Emory University, Atlanta, Georgia, United States of America
[2]Children's Healthcare of Atlanta, Atlanta, Georgia, United States of America
[3]Division of Biostatistics and Bioinformatics, Emory University School of Public Health, Atlanta, Georgia, United States of America
[4]Division of Pediatric Rheumatology, Emory University, Atlanta, Georgia, United States of America

* Correspondence: Catherine Park, MD, Emory University Department of Pediatric Nephrology, 2015 Uppergate Drive NE, Atlanta, GA 30322, United States. Email: catkwpark@gmail.com

ABSTRACT

We enrolled 22 SLE patients (8-19 years old) over three months during clinic visits. Demographic information and medical history were self-reported and collected from medical records. Health and numeracy literacy were assessed using short test of functional health literacy (S-TOFHLA) and Newest Vital Signs (NVS), respectively. Results: Out of the 22 patients, 19 (86%) were female. The greatest percentage by race was Black (45%), and 32% of patients identified as Hispanic. The median age of the participants at the time of the study was 15 years while the median age at diagnosis was 13.5 years. All of the patients surveyed had an adequate score on the S-TOFHLA while only 36% (95% CI: 17.2%-59.3%) scored adequate on the NVS. 27% of the patients surveyed stated that they have been exposed to secondhand smoke, and 9% had tried cigarettes and/or other tobacco products. Conclusion: Although all of the patients surveyed scored adequate levels on the S-TOFHLA, the majority scored in the limited/inadequate range on the numeracy test. This is concerning, as numeracy skills are critical for patients to optimally take medications and follow recommendations including dietary guidelines. Based on these results, going forward, we would like to provide patient recommendations that take into account their numeracy and health literacy levels. One potential way to do this is to create patient education material for easier identification of pills and pill dosages as a first step towards increasing adherence and improving patient outcomes.

INTRODUCTION

Systemic lupus erythematosus (SLE) is a multifactorial autoimmune disease that has the potential to affect multiple organ systems. It affects people of all ages and races, but racial and ethnic minority groups are disproportionately affected with almost double in Black women when compared to White (1-3). Childhood-onset SLE (cSLE) is commonly defined as being diagnosed at <18 years of age, and about 20% of SLE cases present in this age group. Involvement of some organ systems, such as kidneys, have been found to be more common and with higher disease severity in cSLE when compared to adult-onset SLE (4). As of yet, the etiology of SLE is not fully understood. The presumed pathophysiology is that one has a genetic predisposition and then potential factors including environmental stresses, such as smoking, diet, drugs, and hormones trigger the development of SLE (5). Given the variability of symptoms with the common symptoms being nonspecific, such as fatigue, weakness, and joint pains, along with symptom severity ranging from mild to severe, the diagnosis of SLE can be quite challenging. This generally results in a delay in diagnosis of about two years from the onset of symptoms (6, 7). Additionally, achieving favorable long-term outcomes in a disease process that has a severe impact on quality of life can prove to be challenging. Successful long-term outcomes in chronic conditions depend largely on education, awareness, and developing self-management skills, which include administering medications appropriately and consistently, managing symptoms, and navigating the life style changes along with the psychosocial components of one's condition (8, 9).

A major barrier to managing chronic conditions today is non-adherence to medications and other management recommendations (10-12). There is a high prevalence of medication non-adherence in adolescents, which puts them at higher risk for worse outcomes (13). For SLE specifically, medication non-adherence is as high as 40% with a recent study specifically looking at cSLE showing medication non-adherence at 19.7% (14-16). One proposed tool to improve medication adherence is to individualize patient education by focusing on health literacy and providing patient instructions based on health literacy levels. Health literacy is defined as "the capacity to obtain, process, and understand basic health information and services needed to make appropriate health decisions" (17). The 2003 National Assessment of Adult Literacy, which was a seminal study looking at adult literacy levels in the United States, was administered to more than 19,000 individuals aged 16 years and older. This study found that approximately 36% had limited health literacy levels defined as scoring at basic or below basic levels. This study along with several additional analyses of the study showed that factors, such as poverty, race/ethnicity, disability, age, and education, can all influence health literacy levels (HLL) (18, 19). In particular, low HLL along with low literacy in general are associated with lower income and racial/ethnic minority groups (17, 20). This makes it crucial that HLL in disease processes that affect racial/ethnic minority groups more, such as SLE, are assessed. There is growing evidence to suggest that addressing health literacy will have significant benefits in chronic pediatric illness (20, 21).

In addition to reading, numeracy skills are an important variable when it comes to health literacy. Studies have shown that although numeracy skills can be equivalent to literacy skills, many patients actually tend to have poorer quantitative skills (18, 22). A 2018 study done at a single pediatric center looked at health literacy, including numeracy, in pediatric kidney transplant recipients and found that 95% of the patients had adequate literacy skills but only 27% had adequate numeracy skills (23). An adequate functional HLL is crucial to comprehend information provided by healthcare providers and develop lifelong behaviors needed for successful adherence and ultimately favorable long-term outcomes (21, 24-26).

Integrated with traditional health literacy skills is the emerging and evolving field of environmental health literacy, which is defined as "an understanding of the connection between environmental exposures and human health" and its impact on patient outcomes (27). The 2018 data from the National Youth Tobacco Survey showed that the prevalence of tobacco product use was 27.1% in high school students, and 7.2% in middle school students; both were increased when compared to 2017 data (28). Data on secondhand smoke exposure in children showed that the prevalence was more than 37% in 2016 (29-31), and the exposure was highest among those living in poverty as well as among non-Hispanic blacks. Several studies have shown that environmental cigarette smoke is associated with an increased risk of the development of SLE in individuals with a genetic predisposition (32-34). Therefore, in children of a younger age with cSLE, secondhand smoke exposure also needs to be considered as a risk factor for SLE. In a disease process where environmental triggers can potentially worsen outcomes or lead to flares, it is crucial to also increase awareness of environmental health literacy.

The primary aim of this study was to determine the functional HLL, which included literacy, numeracy, and environmental, of cSLE patients in a pediatric center in Atlanta, Georgia where there are about 400 cSLE patients under the combined care of Rheumatology and Nephrology services. We determined if lower HLL were associated with increased healthcare utilization defined as number of Emergency Room (ER) visits and hospitalizations per year. Given previous results for pediatric patients with kidney transplants in the same geographic region, we hypothesize that cSLE patients in this study will have lower HLL, particularly with numeracy literacy. Since understanding of prescriptions is essential in accurately taking medications at home, lower numeracy skills may prove to be a barrier in optimal self-management leading to poorer outcomes, hence we also hypothesize that lower HLL will be associated with increased medical complications and increased healthcare utilization. A secondary aim was to estimate smoking and exposure to secondhand smoke. We hypothesize that the prevalence of secondhand smoke exposure in cSLE patients will be at the least the same or higher than the general population.

OUR STUDY

Approval for this study was obtained through the Institutional Internal Review Board. This was a cross-sectional study and a retrospective chart review over the span of 2 months (2/1/2019-3/31/2019), enrolling 22 SLE patients ranging from 8 to 19 years of age. Demographic information and medical history were collected at the time of scheduled clinic visits. Our primary outcome measures were hospitalizations and ER visits related to SLE.

Inclusion and exclusion criteria

Inclusion criteria for this study were cSLE patients between the ages of 8 and 21 years who speak and understand English. Parents/caretakers/guardians of cSLE patients were also able to participate if they were able to speak, read, and/or understand English. Exclusion criteria were those who could not speak, read, and/or understand English, had cognitive delay, were unable to provide informed consent, and were outside the age range of 8 to 21 years.

Survey design

The Short Test of Functional Health Literacy (S-TOFHLA), a validated measure assessing health literacy (35), and the Newest Vital Signs (NVS), a validated measure assessing numeracy skills (36, 37), were administered during the clinic visit and the results were used to determine baseline functional HLL. Patients were also asked to fill out a secondhand smoke exposure survey, which is adapted from the CDC Youth Tobacco survey, to assess exposure (38). Clinical information was obtained from patient's medical records from the time of SLE diagnosis to the end of the study period (3/31/2019). We used this information to determine a healthcare utilization rate defined as the total number of ER visits and hospitalizations per patient-year.

Data analysis

Based on the results of the S-TOFHLA and NVS, individuals were classified as either having adequate HLL or inadequate HLL with adequate being a score of 23-36 on S-TOFHLA and 4-6 on NVS (35-37). Participants were placed in the inadequate group if they scored in the inadequate/marginal range for the S-TOFHLA (0-16 and 17-22 respectively) or in the inadequate/limited range on the NVS (0-1 and 2-3 respectively). Proportions of adequate/inadequate literacy were calculated with the 95% confidence interval (CI) using the Clopper-Pearson exact method. Fisher's exact test was used for categorical data while Wilcoxon rank sum was used for testing continuous data by adequate vs inadequate groups. Poisson test was used to analyze healthcare utilization between the adequate and inadequate HLL groups. Exact confidence intervals for healthcare utilization were calculated, which is based on the binomial distribution given the small sample size.

FINDINGS

Of the 22 individuals who participated, 86% were female. The greatest percentage in race were Black (45%), while 32% identified themselves as White-Hispanic. The median age of the participants at recruitment was 15 years while the median age at diagnosis was 13.5 years (see Table 1). All of the individuals who participated scored in the adequate range for the S-TOFHLA (see Figure 1). However, for the NVS, only eight patients (36%) scored in the adequate range while the remaining 14 (64%) scored in the inadequate range (combination of high likelihood of limited numeracy skills and possibility of limited numeracy skills) (see figure 2). Of note, we attempted to assess the parents' functional health literacy as well, but due to the scarcity of the responses, found that the data could not be analyzed meaningfully.

Since all participants scored in the adequate range under S-TOFHLA, the individuals were divided into an adequate and inadequate health literacy group based on their NVS scores. Baseline characteristics were compared by health literacy group. There were no statistically significant differences in age, gender, race, ethnicity, and duration of disease between the groups The mean (SD) age in years was 15.4 (2.2) for the inadequate group and 15.3 (2.7) for the adequate group. The mean (SD) age in years at diagnosis for the adequate HLL group was 12.1 (2.2) and 13.5 (1.8) for the inadequate HLL group although this difference was not statistically significant (Table 2). The inadequate HLL group had an average (SD) of 5.71 (6.35) number of hospitalizations/ER visits for the individuals' disease course compared to 5.25 (7.55) per disease course for the adequate HLL group. However, if we take into account the actual duration of illness/follow-up, a significant difference was present between the groups. The eight adequate HLL individuals had a healthcare utilization rate of 1.62 (95% CI 0.14 – 6.61) per patient-year, while the 14 inadequate HLL individuals had a healthcare utilization rate of 3.0 (95% CI 0.63 – 8.80) per patient-year. Therefore, using a Poisson test, a significant difference was detected in healthcare utilization by group (Table 3).

In regard to the secondhand smoke survey, 27% of the individuals surveyed stated that they have been exposed, and 9% reported trying cigarette and/or other tobacco products. Those who reported trying tobacco products stated that they were not exposed to secondhand smoke.

Table 1. Baseline characteristics of the 22 p-SLE participants

Demographics	**p-SLE Patients** **N = 22**
Gender, n (%)	
Female	19 (86%)
Male	3 (14%)
Race, n (%)	
White	9 (41%)
Black	10 (45%)
Asian	3 (14%)
Ethnicity, n (%)	
Hispanic	7 (32%)
Non-Hispanic	15 (68%)
Age at diagnosis (years), median (Q1,Q3)	13.48 (11.94, 14.56)
Duration of disease (months), median (Q1,Q3)	23 (11.04, 46.09)

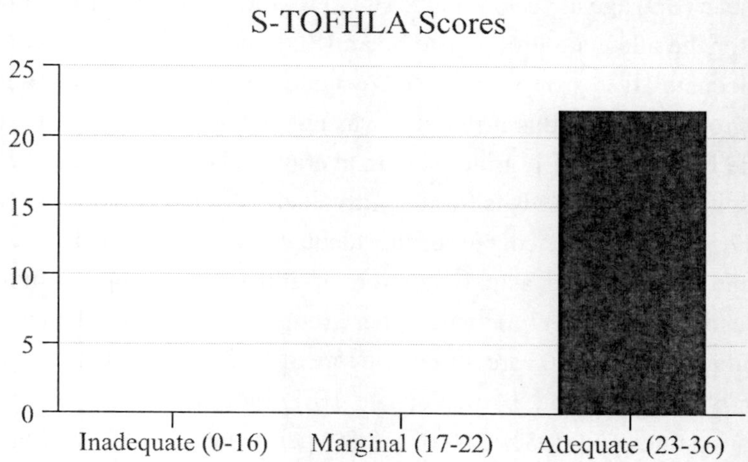

Figure 1. S-TOFHLA scores.

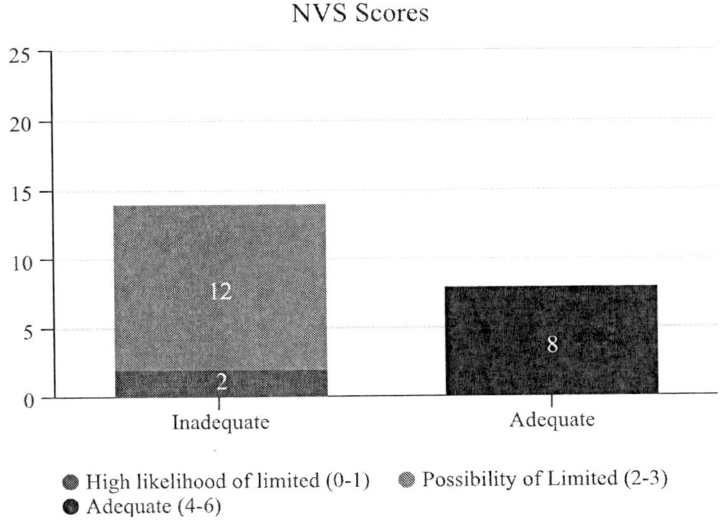

Figure 2. NVS scores.

Table 2. Patient characteristics compared by inadequate and adequate HLL based on scores from newest vital signs (numeracy test)

Variable	Overall (n = 22)	Inadequate HLL (n = 14)	Adequate HLL (n = 8)	p-value
Age, mean (SD)	15.4 (2.3)	15.4 (2.2)	15.3 (2.7)	0.97
Age at diagnosis, mean (SD)	13.0 (2.0)	13.5 (1.8)	12.1 (2.2)	0.15
Gender, n (%)				0.53
Female	19 (86.4)	13 (92.9)	6 (75.0)	
Male	3 (13.6)	1 (7.1)	2 (25.0)	
Race, n (%)				0.69
White	9 (40.9)	6 (42.9)	3 (37.5)	
Black	10 (45.5)	7 (50.0)	3 (37.5)	
Asian	3 (13.6)	1 (7.1)	2 (25.0)	
Ethnicity, n (%)				1.00
Hispanic or Latino	7 (31.8)	4 (28.6)	3 (37.5)	
Non-Hispanic	15 (68.2)	10 (71.4)	5 (62.5)	

Table 3. Healthcare utilization rates compared by inadequate and adequate Hll based on scores from newest vital signs (numeracy test)

	Overall (n = 22)	Inadequate HLL (n = 14)	Adequate HLL (n = 8)	p-value
Duration of illness calculated (yrs), mean (SD)	2.38 (2.19)	1.89 (1.54)	3.24 (2.95)	0.27
Number of hospitalizations or ER visits, mean (SD)	5.55 (6.64)	5.71 (6.35)	5.25 (7.55)	
Healthcare utilization, ER visits/hospitalizations per yr (95% CI)		3.02 (0.63 – 8.80)	1.62 (0.14 – 6.61)	0.0011*

DISCUSSION

To our knowledge, there are a lack of studies looking at functional health literacy in cSLE patients and its effect on clinical outcomes. A few small studies on adult SLE patients show that a low HLL was present in about 20-50% of the population and was associated with worse chronic organ damage and patient reported outcomes (39, 40). Generally, assessing pediatric health literacy can be more complex given the developing literacy skills of pediatric patients along with the need for adequate parent or caregiver's literacy levels. Therefore, health literacy in both the pediatric patients and their caregivers need to be carefully assessed and addressed (41). This is imperative for a disease process that is known to be more prevalent in lower socioeconomic groups since low health literacy is an important underlying factor in further widening the gap in healthcare disparities (42).

The results of this study show that the demographics of our small sample size are similar to previous cSLE studies with the majority of the sample being female and from a racial or ethnic minority group. Although 100% of the individuals surveyed scored at adequate levels on the S-TOFHLA, the majority scored in the limited/inadequate range for their numeracy skills based on the NVS. In an age group where medication adherence is already problematic, these results are concerning. Since SLE is known to affect multiple organ systems, the majority of patients are responsible for managing multiple prescriptions, and numeracy skills are vital in accurately interpreting and optimally adhering to these prescriptions. If an individual also has renal involvement, it is critical to be able to read food labels and determine how much sodium, potassium, and phosphorous are in the foods, which requires adequate numeracy skills.

A recent study in 2018 looked at health literacy disparity and its effect on adolescents and young adults with chronic or end-stage kidney disease (43). Results from this study did not show major differences between low and adequate health literacy groups on healthcare utilization defined as preventable hospitalizations, total hospitalizations, length of hospital stay, and ER visits (43). For the cSLE patients surveyed in our study though the results did indicate that healthcare utilization, defined as ER visits and hospitalizations pertaining to SLE, differed between low and adequate health literacy groups. According to patient reports, SLE has a tremendous impact on the quality of life of patients, caretakers, family members, employment, financial status, and work productivity (44). Therefore, the ultimate goal in SLE management is to get patients on an effective maintenance medication regimen to prevent flares/relapse and eventually improve quality of life for both the child and the family. Our results indicate that the group with inadequate HLL had increased utilization of healthcare services, which suggests an increased risk for worse outcomes.

The estimate of health literacy was the primary focus of this study. Although the utilization rates were not compared for all possible confounders due to small sample size, these results still indicate that the need for counseling and instruction based on one's health literacy level may be an optimal point of intervention to break the cycle of health disparities for children with SLE (see Figure 3). In particular, health literacy interventions

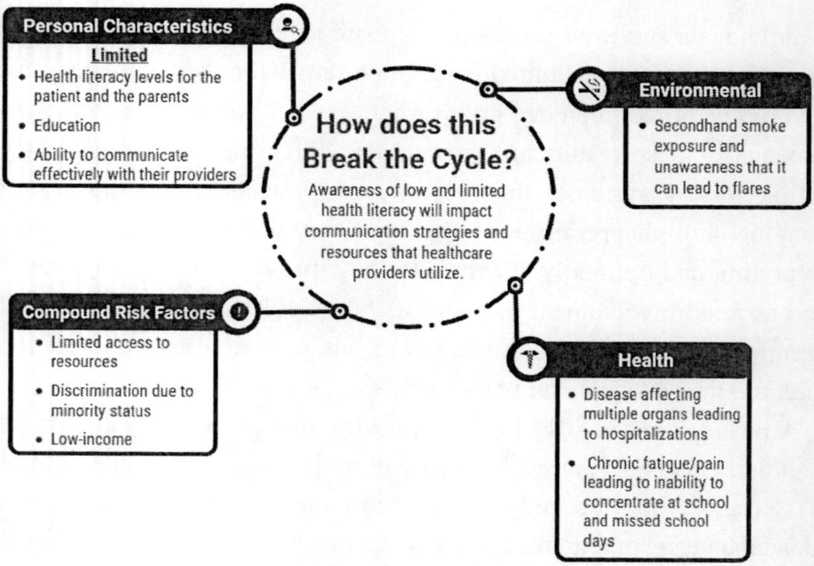

Figure 3. Breaking the cycle of health disparities related to health literacy including numeracy skills and environmental health literacy.

targeting high-risk groups, such as cSLE patients, may improve outcomes and ultimately break the cycle of health disparities. Given SLE affects minority groups more often and a lower socioeconomic status is associated with more severe disease, the cycle of health disparities is perpetuated by resources that may not be appropriate for those with limited education and/or lower HLL. Several resources are available to these patients, either in the form of online material, written pamphlets, or written instructions from the providers, but resources are of limited value if the individual is not able to read, understand, remember, and adequately act on the instructions at home. A recent randomized controlled trial showed a statistically significant and clinically meaningful effect on medication decision making in patients with lupus nephritis when using a computerized decision aid that is individualized and culturally tailored compared to an American College of Rheumatology lupus pamphlet (45). One possible indicator of poor health literacy is identification of pills by the color and size and not by their names. One way to combat misidentification of medications due to the inability to identify them by name is to provide patients with pictures of commonly used SLE medications and demonstrate which pills and how many of them to take (46-48). Studies done in pediatric diabetic patients and parents have shown that hands-on demonstration of how to dose medications have been helpful particularly for individuals with low HLL (49). Another key intervention is the teach-back/show-back method, which has been confirmed in several studies to be highly effective in improving communication and confirming understanding (50-52). Ultimately, our recommendation would be to individualize the education process based on each individual's education status as well as health literacy level.

This study also revealed that about a quarter of the cSLE patients were exposed to secondhand smoke, which is less than the prevalence for the general population. This is interesting given that the cSLE patients tend to have the demographics of individuals with higher risk for secondhand smoke exposure. What the smoking survey was not able to adequately ascertain though was the difficulty that participants had in not fully understanding the concept of secondhand smoke exposure. This observation suggests that, although this was not formally tested, environmental health literacy may be inadequate in this patient population as well as not discussed adequately by the providers. Further evaluation of this along with increased awareness for our patients are needed.

Limitations

One of the major limitations to this study is the small sample size. The majority of the individuals with cSLE were recruited in the general nephrology or rheumatology clinic setting as opposed to in the end-stage renal disease clinics, such as chronic kidney disease, dialysis, and transplant clinics. This could potentially represent a selection bias since the individuals with more significant disease and potentially lower HLL and limited transportation resources may not come to clinic as often. There is also a chance that patients with perceived lower HLL declined to participate due to fear of taking a literacy test although only two patients declined to participate. Another limitation is that this data analysis did not take into account any potential confounders, such as income, education level, minority status, which could affect our results. Furthermore, the ER visits and hospitalizations counted in this study were only those that occurred at our single center so if patients went to other ER's or were hospitalized at other hospitals, they were not counted, which could skew results. Of note, the hospital assessed in this study is the main hospital that provides pediatric rheumatology and nephrology care to the majority of Georgia. Therefore, most of the patients with cSLE in Georgia are likely to attend the clinic at this hospital and are likely to visit this specific hospital's ER, be admitted to this particular hospital, or at least contact the clinic when there is a concern. At this age, some of the medical management is still done by parents, which was not asked in the surveys. If the medical care is strictly managed by the parents or other caregivers, then it is crucial to determine their HLL as well. One of the exclusion criteria in this study was not being able to speak, read, and/or write English; however, the subjects were not asked what the primary language was spoken at home, which could potentially affect literacy levels.

Future directions

Results of this preliminary study were suggestive that HLL can potentially affect one's outcomes. Therefore, the next steps would be to recruit more caregivers if they are doing the majority of the medical management as well as do further data analyses to account for the aforementioned limitations. The take-home message is to focus the efforts on individualizing the education process, and in turn, improve communication between the providers and the patients with lower HLL. One plan for the future is two-tiered. The goal is to increase awareness amongst the providers about the potential for patients to have limited HLL as well as create optimal educational materials for our cSLE patients for easier identification of medications so that they can successfully demonstrate the teach-back method. These interventions can ultimately improve home management and aide patients in decreasing medical complications and potentially achieving better quality of life and thus break the cycle of health disparities for children with SLE.

ACKNOWLEDGMENTS

This research was supported by the Emory University Department of Pediatrics and Children's Healthcare of Atlanta.

REFERENCES

[1] Kamphuis S, Silverman ED. Prevalence and burden of pediatric-onset systemic lupus erythematosus. Nat Rev Rheumatol 2010;6(9):538-46.

[2] Hiraki LT, Benseler SM, Tyrrell PN, Harvey E, Hebert D, Silverman ED. Ethnic differences in pediatric systemic lupus erythematosus. J Rheumatol 2009;36(11):2539-46.

[3] Feldman CH, Hiraki LT, Liu J, Fischer MA, Solomon DH, Alarcon GS, et al. Epidemiology and sociodemographics of systemic lupus erythematosus and lupus nephritis among US adults with Medicaid coverage, 2000-2004. Arthritis Rheum 2013;65(3):753-63.

[4] Tarr T, Dérfalvi B, Gyori N, Szántó A, Siminszky Z, Malik A, et al. Similarities and differences between pediatric and adult patients with systemic lupus erythematosus. Lupus 2015;24(8):796-803.

[5] Somers E, Richardson B. Environmental exposures, epigenetic changes and the risk of lupus. Lupus 2014;23(6):568-76.

[6] Moriarty T, O'Sullivan M, Tam A, Goncalves RM, Wall JG. Systemic lupus erythematosus in Portugal: diagnosis and disease awareness from 1970 to 2001. Eur J Epidemiol 2003;18(10):995-9.

[7] Gergianaki I, Bertsias G. Systemic lupus erythematosus in primary Care: An update and practical messages for the general practitioner. Front Med (Lausanne) 2018;5:16 .

[8] Barlow J, Wright C, Sheasby J, Turner A, Hainsworth J. Self-mancagement approaches for people with chronic conditions: A review. Patient Educ Cours 2002;48(2):177-87.

[9] Scalzi LV, Hollenbeak CS, Mascuilli E, Olsen N. Improvement of medication adherence in adolescents and young adults with SLE using web-based education with and without a social media intervention, a pilot study. Pediatr Rheumatol Online J 2018;16(1):18.

[10] Sokol MC, McGuigan KA, Verbrugge RR, Epstein RS. Impact of medication adherence on hospitalization risk and healthcare cost. Med Care 2005;43(6):521-30.

[11] Kleinsinger F. The Unmet Challenge of Medication Nonadherence. Perm J 2018;22:18-033.

[12] Cutler RL, Fernandez-Llimos F, Frommer M, Benrimoj C, Garcia-Cardenas V. Economic impact of medication non-adherence by disease groups: A systematic review. BMJ Open 2018;8(1):e016982.

[13] Taddeo D, Egedy M, Frappier JY. Adherence to treatment in adolescents. Paediatr Child Health 2008;13(1):19-24.

[14] Koneru S, Shishov M, Ware A, Farhey Y, Mongey AB, Graham TB, et al. Effectively measuring adherence to medications for systemic lupus erythematosus in a clinical setting. Arthritis Rheum 2007;57(6):1000-6.

[15] Daleboudt GM, Broadbent E, McQueen F, Kaptein AA. Intentional and unintentional treatment nonadherence in patients with systemic lupus erythematosus. Arthritis Care Res (Hoboken) 2011;63(3):342-50.

[16] Davis AM, Graham TB, Zhu Y, McPheeters ML. Depression and medication nonadherence in childhood-onset systemic lupus erythematosus. Lupus 2018;27(9):1532-41.

[17] Nielsen-Bohlman L, Panzer AM, Kindig DA, eds. Health literacy: A prescription to end Confusion. Washington, DC: National Academies Press, 2004.

[18] Kutner M GE, Jin Y, Paulsen C. The health literacy of America's adults: Results from the 2003 National Assessment of Adult Literacy. Washington, DC: National Center for Education Statistics, 2006.

[19] Rikard RV, Thompson MS, McKinney J, Beauchamp A. Examining health literacy disparities in the United States: A third look at the National Assessment of Adult Literacy (NAAL). BMC Public Health 2016;16(1):975.

[20] Sanders LM, Shaw JS, Guez G, Baur C, Rudd R. Health literacy and child health promotion: implications for research, clinical care, and public policy. Pediatrics 2009;124(Suppl 3):S306-14.

[21] Morrison AK, Glick A, Yin HS. Health literacy: Implications for child health. Pediatr Rev 2019;40(6):263-77.

[22] Rothman RL, Montori VM, Cherrington A, Pignone MP. Perspective: The role of numeracy in health care. J Health Commun 2008;13(6):583-95.

[23] Kamel M MC, Wilkerson A, Alexander N, Gazmararian J, George R. Effects of health literacy and numeracy literacy on adherence, quality of life and readiness to transition in pediatric renal transplant recipients. American Transplant Congress, Seattle, WA, 2018.

[24] Osterberg L, Blaschke T. Adherence to medication. N Engl J Med 2005;353(5): 487-97.

[25] Haynes RB, Yao X, Degani A, Kripalani S, Garg A, McDonald HP. Interventions to enhance medication adherence. Cochrane Database Syst Rev 2005;4:CD000011.

[26] Burkhart PV, Sabate E. Adherence to long-term therapies: evidence for action. J Nurs Scholarsh 2003;35(3):207.

[27] Finn S, O'Fallon L. The emergence of environmental health literacy-from its roots to its future potential. Environ Health Perspect 2017;125(4):495-501.

[28] Gentzke AS, Creamer M, Cullen KA, Ambrose BK, Willis G, Jamal A, et al. Vital signs: Tobacco product use among middle and high school students - United States, 2011-2018. MMWR 2019;68(6):157-64.

[29] Merianos AL, Jandarov RA, Mahabee-Gittens EM. Secondhand smoke exposure and pediatric healthcare visits and hospitalizations. Am J Prev Med 2017;53(4):441-8.

[30] Homa DM, Neff LJ, King BA, Caraballo RS, Bunnell RE, Babb SD, et al. Vital signs: disparities in nonsmokers' exposure to secondhand smoke--United States, 1999-2012. MMWR 2015;64(4):103-8.

[31] Tsai J, Homa DM, Gentzke AS, Mahoney M, Sharapova SR, Sosnoff CS, et al. Exposure to secondhand smoke among nonsmokers - United States, 1988-2014. MMWR 2018;67(48):1342-6.

[32] Takvorian SU, Merola JF, Costenbader KH. Cigarette smoking, alcohol consumption and risk of systemic lupus erythematosus. Lupus 2014;23(6):537-44.

[33] Costenbader KH, Kim DJ, Peerzada J, Lockman S, Nobles-Knight D, Petri M, et al. Cigarette smoking and the risk of systemic lupus erythematosus: a meta-analysis. Arthritis Rheum 2004;50(3):849-57.

[34] Barbhaiya M, Costenbader KH. Environmental exposures and the development of systemic lupus erythematosus. Curr Opin Rheumatol 2016;28(5):497-505.

[35] Baker DW, Williams MV, Parker RM, Gazmararian JA, Nurss J. Development of a brief test to measure functional health literacy. Patient Educ Couns 1999;38(1): 33-42.

[36] Weiss BD, Mays MZ, Martz W, Castro KM, DeWalt DA, Pignone MP, et al. Quick assessment of literacy in primary care: the newest vital sign. Ann Fam Med 2005;3(6):514-22.

[37] Housten AJ, Lowenstein LM, Hoover DS, Leal VB, Kamath GR, Volk RJ. Limitations of the S-TOFHLA in measuring poor numeracy: a cross-sectional study. BMC Public Health 2018;18(1):405.

[38] National Youth Tobacco Survey (NYTS). URL: https://dataverse.harvard.edu/dataset.xhtml?persistentId=doi:10.7910/DVN/UX2FPT.

[39] Marengo MF KM, De Achaval S, Cox V, Garcia A, Richardson M, Suarez-Almazor ME. Impact of health literacy on treatment adherence and clinical outcomes in patients with systemic lupus erythematosus. American College of Rheumatology, Chicago, Illinois, 2011.

[40] Katz PP DEM, Trupin L, Lanata C, Rush S, Helmick CG, Criswell LA, Yazdany J. The impact of limited health literacy on patient-reported outcomes (PROs) in systemic lupus erythematosus (SLE). American College of Rheumatology Annual Meeting, San Diego, CA, 2017.

[41] Sanders LM, Federico S, Klass P, Abrams MA, Dreyer B. Literacy and child health: A systematic review. Arch Pediatr Adolesc Med 2009;163(2):131-40.

[42] Mantwill S, Monestel-Umana S, Schulz PJ. The relationship between health literacy and health disparities: A systematic review. PLoS One 2015;10(12):e0145455.

[43] Levine R, Javalkar K, Nazareth M, Faldowski RA, de Ferris MD, Cohen S, et al. Disparities in health literacy and healthcare utilization among adolescents and young adults with chronic or end-stage kidney disease. J Pediatr Nurs 2018;38:57-61.

[44] Kent T, Davidson A, Newman D, Buck G, D'Cruz D. Burden of illness in systemic lupus erythematosus: Results from a UK patient and carer online survey. Lupus 2017;26(10):1095-100.

[45] Singh JA, Fraenkel L, Green C, Alarcon GS, Barton JL, Saag KG, et al. Individualized decision aid for diverse women with lupus nephritis (IDEA-WON): A randomized controlled trial. PLoS Med 2019;16(5):e1002800.

[46] McMahon SR, Rimsza ME, Bay RC. Parents can dose liquid medication accurately. Pediatrics 1997;100(3 Pt 1):330-3.

[47] Yin HS, Dreyer BP, van Schaick L, Foltin GL, Dinglas C, Mendelsohn AL. Randomized controlled trial of a pictogram-based intervention to reduce liquid medication dosing errors and improve adherence among caregivers of young children. Arch Pediatr Adolesc Med 2008;162(9):814-22.

[48] Dowse R, Ehlers M. Medicine labels incorporating pictograms: do they influence understanding and adherence? Patient Educ Couns 2005;58(1):63-70.

[49] Howe CJ, Cipher DJ, LeFlore J, Lipman TH. Parent health literacy and communication with diabetes educators in a pediatric diabetes clinic: A mixed methods approach. J Health Commun 2015;20(Suppl 2):50-9.

[50] Griffey RT, Shin N, Jones S, Aginam N, Gross M, Kinsella Y, et al. The impact of teach-back on comprehension of discharge instructions and satisfaction among emergency patients with limited health literacy: A randomized, controlled study. J Commun Healthcare 2015;8(1):10-21.

[51] Badaczewski A, Bauman LJ, Blank AE, Dreyer B, Abrams MA, Stein REK, et al. Relationship between Teach-back and patient-centered communication in primary care pediatric encounters. Patient Educ Couns 2017;100(7):1345-52.

[52] Wolf MS, Davis TC, Shrank W, Rapp DN, Bass PF, Connor UM, et al. To err is human: Patient misinterpretations of prescription drug label instructions. Patient Educ Couns 2007;67(3):293-300.

In: Child Environmental Health Disparities ISBN: 978-1-53617-823-4
Editors: IL Rubin and J Merrick

Chapter 10

DID MEDICAID EXPANSION DECREASE DISPARITIES FOR RECEIPT OF PREVENTIVE MEDICAL CARE AMONG VULNERABLE CHILDREN?

Patricia Daniel[1,*], PhD, Audrey Leroux[2], PhD and Brian Barger[1], PhD

[1]Center for Leadership in Disability, Georgia State University and
[2]Department of Educational Policy Studies, Georgia State University, Atlanta, Georgia, United States of America

ABSTRACT

In this chapter we investigate differences in receipt of pediatric preventive medical visits (PMV) among racial/ethnic groups between the states that did and did not expand Medicaid as a part of the 2010 Affordable Care Act. Differences were investigated using hierarchical linear modeling. Tested models included whether respondents were first generation immigrant families, if English was spoken in the home, whether the child had special

---

* Corresponding Author's email: pdmath@yahoo.com.

health care needs, if there was an insurance gap, and race/ethnicity of the child as level-1 variables and residence state as a level-2 variable to predict odds ratios of PMV, with cross-level interactions between race/ethnicity and Medicaid expansion. All groups of children living in states with Medicaid expansion had increased log-odds of receiving a PMV. When the interactions between race/ethnicity and Medicaid expansion were considered, the odds of PMV among Whites, Hispanics, Black, and other race/ethnicity children was greater in Medicaid expansion states; however, the strongest effect was for White children. If the interaction term was not considered, children of Hispanic and Other ethnicity had significantly lower odds of receiving PMV in both expansion and non-expansion states. Children who did not speak English in the home, were first generation immigrant families, and/or experienced a gap in insurance had reduced odds ratios for receiving PMV compared to other children.

INTRODUCTION

The Affordable Care Act of 2010 (ACA) was introduced to improve health care coverage for United States citizens. The ACA included a goal to expand Medicaid to cover all families below 138% of the poverty level (1), but not all states opted to expand Medicaid coverage. Medicaid is a public health insurance program, funded by a combination of federal and state monies. Both federal and state funds are managed by the states, resulting in many different approaches to administering Medicaid (1). Prior to 2014 the median income to qualify for Medicaid was $15,000 for a family of four, with wide variation from state to state. Children's health benefits were mandated by the federal government through the Children's Health Insurance Program (CHIP) program for children whose family income fell below 100% federal poverty level, $23,842 for a family of four (1). After 2014 the median income for a family of four qualifying for Medicaid rose to $33,465. All states lost federal funding for uncompensated healthcare as part of the ACA, but these losses were expected to be balanced with a greater proportion of healthcare costs paid through Medicaid (1, 2). As funds for uncompensated care were reduced--in all states--the number of people covered by Medicaid did not increase, but decreased in non-expanded states, due to changes in waiver legislation. The states that did not expand lost a large portion of their federal funding for healthcare (2). The monies that had been flowing to uncompensated health care were diverted to Medicaid, so if a state did not expand Medicaid, it generally lost funding.

While the ACA expansion was primarily aimed at adults, the fact that children follow their caretakers into insurance coverage suggests that children should reap benefits as well (3). It is reasonable to expect that the Medicaid expansion increased children's access to health care. One important outcome of Medicaid expansion is whether children have increased access to a preventive medical visit (PMV), an indicator of children's access to preventive health care (4). Preventive health care is important for connecting children to health care providers who promote health, teach caretakers and children to make better health decisions, and help prevent and/or detect disease early (5). During a preventive health visit children and caretakers receive guidance in promoting physical, emotional, and intellectual development. This help includes guidance to choose appropriate nutrition, exercise, and safety habits such as car seat and helmet usage (6); talking and reading to promote intellectual development (7); education and interventions to prevent or reduce adverse childhood events (8), and screening for developmental delays and behavior (5). Further, during these visits children receive vaccinations to prevent disease and reduce health care costs over time (9)

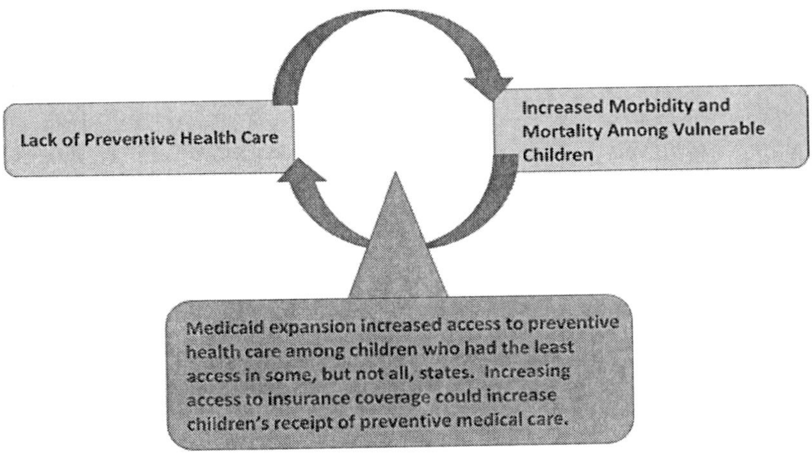

Figure 1. Breaking the cycle of children's environmental health disparities.

Thus, children who receive preventive health care are also less likely to experience preventable illness and more likely to receive timely intervention for health conditions that are not preventable (5). Timely intervention often reduces morbidity and mortality, allowing children longer life spans (5). Thus, PMVs are an important outcome to consider in relation to the ACA Medicaid expansion. Reducing disparities in PMV can break the cycle of environmental health disparities by reducing the disproportionately negative effects of both social and physical determinants of health to which vulnerable children are exposed (see Figure 1).

Medicaid expansion and health disparities

Health disparities among children in the USA are well documented (10). Children of minority race or ethnicity had less desirable health outcomes on many measures including less access to care, lower quality care, and greater morbidity and mortality from disease (11,12). These inequities existed in preventive health care (10) even as preventive care was being promoted to reduce health disparities and reduce health care cost in the US (13).

The ACA is seen as successful in certain respects, as large disparities in healthcare insurance coverage found prior to the ACA were reduced after Medicaid expansion among all racial and ethnic groups, although not equally among all groups (14). Research concerning children's healthcare outcomes in states with Medicaid expansion includes findings of decreased infant mortality (15), reduced disparities in trauma care in adolescents (16), increased school readiness (17), and increased access to mental health care for youth (18). Studies indicate that Medicaid expansion is associated with increased adult preventive care (19) and that there is an increased likelihood of a well child visit among children of low income parents in states with increased eligibility for Medicaid, i.e., as the threshold for Medicaid eligibility is reduced by increasing percent of federal poverty level for eligibility, the probability of a well child visit increases (20). In the study by Venkataramani et al. (20) the data source was 2001-2009 Medical

Expenditure Panel Surveys, thus it does not address differences related to ACA Medicaid expansion.

Factors affecting pediatric health care utilization

There are many factors affecting health care utilization. For example, Anderson's Model of Health Care Consumption (21) suggests that health care consumption is predicted by need, access, and predisposing variables. Predisposing variables include demographics such as age, race, language, income, caretakers' education, family structure, and beliefs; need variables include children with special health care needs (CSHCN) that are more than the health care needs of typically developing children; access variables include health insurance, prior use of the healthcare system, and geographic location (22). Researchers suggest that language can influence a caretaker's assessment of care quality and trust, informing their decision to take a child to a well care provider (23). Also immigrants use less preventive health services than natives (24). Furthermore, community poverty is associated with the emergence of health service "deserts", medically underserved areas or populations, where there are limited healthcare services (25).

Research questions

In the current climate of debate concerning the efficacy of the ACA and Medicaid expansion it is important to determine what, if any, impact Medicaid expansion had on the health care outcomes of US citizens. Our study's goal is to compare the receipt of preventive medical visits among children who lived in states that did, and did not, expand Medicaid.

This study focused on the question: Are children of all races and ethnicities living in Medicaid expansion states more likely to receive preventive health care than in non-expansion states? This study aimed to determine if (a) there are differences among states in the likelihood of receiving a preventive medical visit, (b) if these differences can be attributed to Medicaid expansion, and (c) if disparities among groups of racial and ethnic children's receipt of PMV persist after Medicaid expansion.

Table1. Number of children sampled in each state

State	N	State	N	State	N	State	N
AL	830	IL	1115	MT	1018	RI	893
AK	823	IN	942	NE	1073	SC	885
AZ	887	IO	1132	NV	774	SD	1133
AR	829	KS	1007	NH	995	TN	885
CA	942	KY	879	NJ	1081	TX	813
CO	1101	LA	687	NM	792	UT	1148
CT	1090	MA	986	NY	950	VT	1117
DE	918	MD	1095	NC	951	VA	1158
DC	1001	MA	1185	ND	1051	WA	1141
FL	905	MI	1127	OH	1027	WV	785
GA	795	MN	1351	OK	764	WI	1267
HI	1122	MS	638	OR	1107	WY	835
ID	1068	MO	1015	PA	1099		

Total sample size of individuals = 50,212.

Total number of clusters = 51.

OUR STUDY

The data source was the 2016 National Survey of Children's Health (NSCH), a cross-sectional survey conducted by the US Census Bureau (4). This survey is used to assess the physical and mental well-being of US children ages 0-17 years. A caregiver responded to inquiries focused on the health and health care of one child living in the household in 50,212 randomly selected households (4). Table 1 contains the distribution of the sampled children among the states. Most questions required either a yes/no or a categorical response. The data source for statewide policies was the National Council of State Legislators' database of state legislation (26). The measurement was whether the state did or did not participate in Medicaid expansion before 2016.

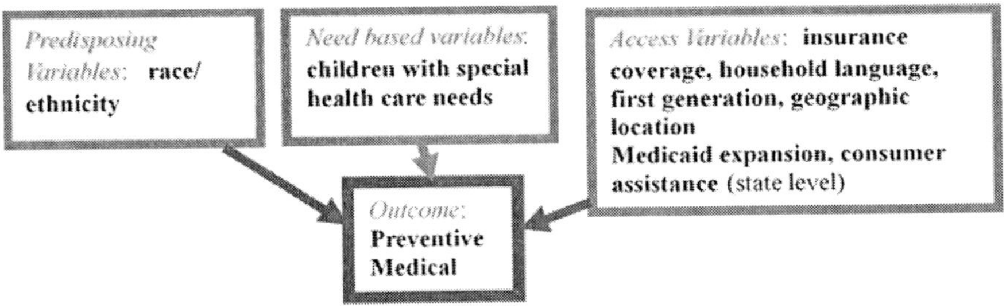

Figure 2. Anderson's model of health care consumption. Anderson (Andersen RM. Revisiting the behavioral model and access to medical care: Does it matter? J Health Soc Behav 1995;36(1):1–10) suggested three types of variables predict health care consumption, predisposing, need based, and access. Our model is focused on the interaction between predisposing variables of race/ethnicity and access increased by living in a Medicaid expanded state.

Outcome and predictors

The outcome variable PMV was the caregiver's yes or no response to the question "Did the child receive one or more PMV in the last 12 months". 433 children (0.8%) were missing the outcome variable, PMV, and their data was deleted from the analysis during model building.

Andersen's model of health care utilization (21) was used to select predictor variables, illustrated in figure 2. The predisposing variables included were speaking English in the home, first generation immigrant families, and race/ethnicity. These choices were based on the research question connecting persistent disparities to Medicaid expansion. The need variable was CSHCN, this is the 2016 NSCH indicator for children who need more healthcare than typical children. Caretakers responded to a series of questions that screened the child as CSHCN or not according to the criteria estimated by the Maternal Child Health Bureau (4). Access variables were insurance gap and state of residence, insurance gap indicating if the child was insured the full 12 months prior to the survey, and state of residence indicating if the child was living in a state that did or did not expand Medicaid.

Immigration and language have been identified in other studies as predictors of PMV (11, 23) suggesting that first generation (family) and English speaking in the home might be significant predictors for this study. The focus of this research was on disparities among race/ ethnic groups. Prior studies have shown that poverty level, family structure and parental education are correlated to race/ethnicity and these are important demographic factors associated with the impact of the ACA (27). We chose race/ethnicity as predictors over the other characteristics as recent research on adults indicates that that the ACA expansion has benefited White populations to a greater degree than other minority groups (14). We included insurance gap in the prior year because Medicaid expansion is aimed at increasing health insurance coverage within the states' populations. Medicaid expansion, the only level-2 (state level) predictor, is a state level policy that may help determine the child's access to health insurance.

The outcome and predictor variables were coded as follows: Children who received PMV were coded PMV = 1, children who did not receive PMV were coded PMV = 0; children who spoke English in the home were coded English = 0, children who did not were coded English = 1; children who were not first generation were coded FirstGen = 0, children who were first generation were coded FirstGen =1. The race/ethnicity indicator in the 2016 NSCH has four categories: Black, Hispanic, Other, and White. Each child is assigned to only one of these categories in the survey. Children who were categorized as Hispanic were coded Hispanic = 1, all other children were coded Hispanic =0; children who were categorized as Black were coded Black = 1, all other children were coded Black = 0; children who were categorized as Other were coded Other =1, all other children were coded Other =0; children who were categorized as White were coded Hispanic =0, Black =0, and Other = 0, making White the reference group for the race/ethnicity variable. Children identified as CSHCN in the survey were coded CSHCN = 1, other children were coded CSHCN =0. Children who experienced an insurance gap in the prior 12 months were coded Gap = 1, other children were coded gap =0. The states that expanded Medicaid were coded Exp = 1, the other states were coded Exp =0.

A cross-level interaction was included in the final model to study the interaction between race and Medicaid expansion among the states. The cross-level interaction was added to the level-2 model for Hispanic, Black, and Other.

Analysis

A Hierarchical Generalized Linear Regression (HGLM) model was built using HLM 7.03 (28). HLM software uses a Bernoulli link function and penalized quasi-likelihood estimation method to produce log-odds of PMV. The unconditional model, predicting the log-odds of an average child in the study receiving PMV with no predictor other than state, separated the model variance into individual variance within the states and state level variance between the states. This model produced an intraclass correlation coefficient of .04, suggesting that 4% of variance was related to state differences, and that a hierarchical modeling approach was appropriate for this study.

Variables in the model were uncentered and all slopes fixed because 51 clusters were too few to allow for random slopes. The model was constructed without interaction terms, and then with cross-level interaction terms for the variables first generation, non-English in the home, Black, Hispanic and other. The interaction terms for first generation and non-English in the home were not significant. The interaction terms for Black, Hispanic, and Other were significant. The final model was built including only interaction terms for the set of race/ethnicity variables, Black, Hispanic, and Other. The final fully conditional model was:

$$\ln\left(\frac{\Pr(PMV_{ij}=1)}{1-\Pr(PMV_{ij}=1)}\right) = \beta_{0j} + \beta_{1j}(English) + \beta_{2j}(FirstGen) + \beta_{3j}(Gap) + \beta_{4j}Hispanic_{ij} + \beta_{5j}Black_{ij} + \beta_{6j}Other_{ij} + \beta_{7j}CSHCN_{ij}$$

$$\beta_{0j} = \gamma_{00} + \gamma_{01}Exp_j + u_{0j}\ ;u_{0j} \sim N\ (0, \tau_{00})$$

$$\beta_{1j} = \gamma_{10}$$

$$\beta_{2j} = \gamma_{20}$$

$$\beta_{3j} = \gamma_{30}$$
$$\beta_{4j} = \gamma_{40} + \gamma_{41}(Exp_j)$$
$$\beta_{5j} = \gamma_{50} + \gamma_{51}(Exp_j)$$
$$\beta_{6j} = \gamma_{60} + \gamma_{61}(Exp_j)$$
$$\beta_{7j} = \gamma_{70};$$

In this model γ_{00} was the expected log-odds of having a PMV for a referent child described as one who: (a) speaks English in the home, (b) is not first generation, (c) had no insurance gap, (d) is White race, (e) does not have special health care needs and (f) lives in a state without Medicaid expansion. γ_{01} represents the expected log-odds of having a PMV in a state that has Medicaid expansion compared to the log-odds in a state that does not, holding all other variables constant. The $\text{gamma}_{10,\ 20,\ 30,40,50,\ 60,\ \text{and}\ 70}$ estimates represent changes in log-odds--controlling for other variables in the model—among children different from the reference group in each predictor category, that is a child who (a) does not speak English in the home, and/or (b) is first generation, and/or (c) had an insurance gap, and/or (d) is of Black, Hispanic, and/or Other race/ethnicity, and/or (e) has special health care needs.

Assumption checking

Assumptions underpinning the use of a 2-level binomial model were checked to determine if this set of predictors and outcome were appropriate for use in HGLM. Pearson correlations among the level-1 predictors and level-1 residuals were calculated and the level-1 predictors were determined to be independent of the level-1 residuals. Pearson correlations among the level-1 predictors were determined and the only highly correlated pair was not speaking English in the home and Hispanic. Not speaking English in the home and Hispanic had a .46 correlation, but both predictors were included because the literature search suggested parental language as an important predictor of PMV (11), and race/ethnicity form the research questions. The level-2 residuals were reasonably normal. There was no correlation between level-2 residuals and level-2 predictors, suggesting independence. There was no correlation between level-1 residuals and level-2 residuals, suggesting they were also independent. The omitted level-1 predictors of poverty level, sex, age, and family structure were not correlated to the level-2 residual.

Table 2. Characteristics of population estimated by the sample

Variable	Sample N	Level	Estimated Population N	Proportion	SE
Preventive Medical Visit	42344	Outcome	59647331	0.81	0.001
No Preventive Medical Visit	7435	Outcome	12858597	0.18	0.001
Medicaid Expansion States	27	2	27	0.54	0.07
Non-Medicaid Expansion States	23	2	23	0.46	0.07
English Speaking in the home	46687	1	6216651	.86	0.001
Not English Speaking in the home	3148	1	695454	.10	0.001
First Generation	8486	1	1876126	0.03	0.001
Not First Generation	39273	1	64749922	.89	0.001
Insurance Gap	2504	1	5882311	0.08	0.001
No Insurance Gap	47708	1	66670823	0.91	0.001
Hispanic ethnicity*	5523	1	18000627	0.25	0.001
Not Hispanic ethnicity	44689	1	55349413	0.75	0.001
Black race*	2871	1	9324320	0.13	0.001
Not Black race	47341	1	64025720	0.87	0.001
Other race*	6501	1	7965888	0.11	0.001
Not Other race	43711	1	65384152	0.89	0.001
Special Health Care Needs	11392	1	14196961	0.19	0.001
No Special Health Care Needs	38820	1	59153079	0.81	0.001

FINDINGS

Population estimates, shown in table 2, were found for the proportions of children with the outcome and predictor variables included in the model. The questions concerning first generation and language spoken in the home had a higher rate of missing responses than other predictors, eight percent and four percent, respectively. All other variables had less than one percent missing responses. 81% of all children were estimated to have received a preventive medical visit in the previous 12 months. An estimated 86% of children spoke English in the home, 10% did not speak English in the home and 4% of respondents did not answer this question. An estimated 89% of respondents said the child being surveyed was not first-generation, 3% of caregivers responded that the child in the survey was first-generation, and 8% of the caregivers did not answer this question. An estimated 91% of children did not experience an insurance gap in the 12 months preceding the survey, 8% did experience an insurance gap. 19% of children were estimated to have a special health care need, 81% did not have a special health care need. Twenty-six of the states included in the 2016 NSCH states expanded Medicaid prior to data collection in 2016.

Table 3. HLM model predicting primary medical visit in the last year of children 0-17 in National Survey of Children's Health (2016)

Fixed Effect	**Coefficient**	**Odds Ratio Ratio**	**Confidence Interval Interval**
For Intercept 1, β_0			
INTRCPT2, γ_{00}	1.62	5.05	(4.48,5.69)
EXP, γ_{01}	0.42	1.53	(1.24,1.88)
For CSHCN slope β_6			
INTRCPT2, γ_{70}	0.54	1.72	(1.59,1.86)
For FIRSTGEN slope, β_1			
INTRCPT2, γ_{10}	-0.45	0.64	(0.45,0.89)
For ENGLISH slope, β_7			
INTRCPT2, γ_{70}	-0.48	0.62	(0.50,0.75)
For GAP slope, β_2			
INTRCPT2, γ_{20}	-0.46	0.63	(0.53,0.75)
For HISPANIC slope, β_3			
INTRCPT2, γ_{30}	-0.07	0.93	(0.80,1.09)
EXP, γ_{31}	-0.19	0.83	(0.68,1.01)
For BLACK slope, β_4			
INTRCPT2, γ_{40}	-0.01	0.98	(0.77,1.25)
EXP, γ_{41}	-0.31	0.73	(0.54,1.03)
For OTHER slope, β_5			
INTRCPT2, γ_{50}	0.05	1.05	(0.91,1.21)
EXP, γ_{51}	-0.26	0.77	(0.64,0.94)

Only fixed effects are reported in this table because there are no random slopes in the final model.

Results of model building

Results of HGLM analysis suggested that children living in Medicaid Expansion states and children with special health care needs were more likely to receive PMV than children who did not live in expanded states and/or who did not have special health care needs, as shown in table 3. The odds ratio for PMV among children in expanded states was 1.53, 95% CI = [1.26, 1.86] times those of children in non-Medicaid expansion states. The odds ratio for PMV among children with special health care needs was 1.72, 95% CI = [1.59,1.86] times those of children who did not have special health care needs.

Several predictors in the model reduced children's odds ratios for PMV. These were first generation, insurance gap, and not speaking English in the home. Odds of PMV among first generation children were 0.64, 95% CI = [0.45, 0.89] times those who were not first generation, odds of PMV among children who experienced an insurance gap in the prior 12 months were 0.63, 95% CI [0.53, 0.75] times those of children who did not experience an insurance gap, and odds of PMV among children who did not speak English in the home were 0.62, 95% CI [0.25, 0.75] times those of children who spoke English in the home.

The race/ethnicity variables were analyzed with cross-level interaction terms added to the final model. The coefficient for cross-level interaction for other was -.26, p-value = .009; the cross-level interaction coefficient for Hispanic was -0.19, p-value = .06, and the cross level interaction coefficient for Black was -0.30, p-value = .05.

Figure 3 is a chart showing the odds ratios for all four race/ethnicity categories in Medicaid expansion states and non-Medicaid expansion states including the interaction between Medicaid expansion and race/ethnicity. The negative interaction coefficients in table 3 suggested that non-White children in Medicaid expansion states had lower odds of PMV than children who were White, but children in all four race/ethnicity categories had increased odds of PMV in Medicaid expansion states versus non-Medicaid expansion states.

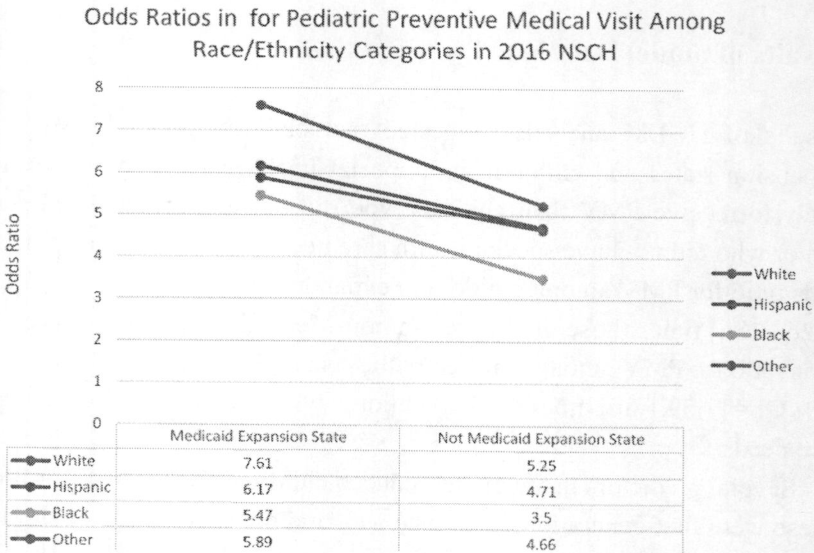

Figure 3. Odds Ratios for PMV produced by the model including interactions between Medicaid expansion and race/ethnicity.
The graph illustrates the negative interaction between Hispanic, Black, and Other race/ethnicities in Medicaid expansion states—the odds ratio for White children is noticeably higher than the other three. The coefficients for the Hispanic and Black race/ethnicity are not statistically significant, the coefficient for Other is statistically significant. The slopes for White and Black are greater than Other and Hispanic, suggesting that Medicaid expansion had a greater impact on White and Black children's receipt of PMV.

Holding all other variables constant, the equation for determining the effects of Medicaid expansion among the race/ethnic groups is:

$$\ln\left(\frac{\Pr(PMV_{ij}=1)}{1-\Pr(PMV_{ij}=1)}\right) = \gamma_{00} + \gamma_{30}(\text{Hispanic}) + \gamma_{40}(\text{Black}) + \gamma_{50}(\text{Other}) + \gamma_{01}(\text{Exp}) + \gamma_{31}(\text{Hispanic})*(\text{Exp}) + \gamma_{41}(\text{Black})*(\text{Exp}) + \gamma_{51}(\text{Other})*(\text{Exp})$$

The race/ethnicities were dummy coded, with White as a reference group. Substituting ones for the desired race and zeros for the other races determined the log-odds for PMV among the group of interest. The log-odds for White children is simply $\gamma_{00.} + \gamma_{01}(\text{Exp})$. In this equation the odds ratio of

White children receiving PMV in Medicaid expansion states was 7.61, in non-expansion states it was 5.25. The odds ratio of Hispanic children receiving PMV in Medicaid expansion states was 6.17, in non-expansion states it was 4.48. The odds ratio of Black children receiving PMV in expansion states was 5.47, in non-expansion states it was 4.50. The odds ratio of Other children receiving PMV in expansion states was 5.89, in non-expansion states it was 4.85.

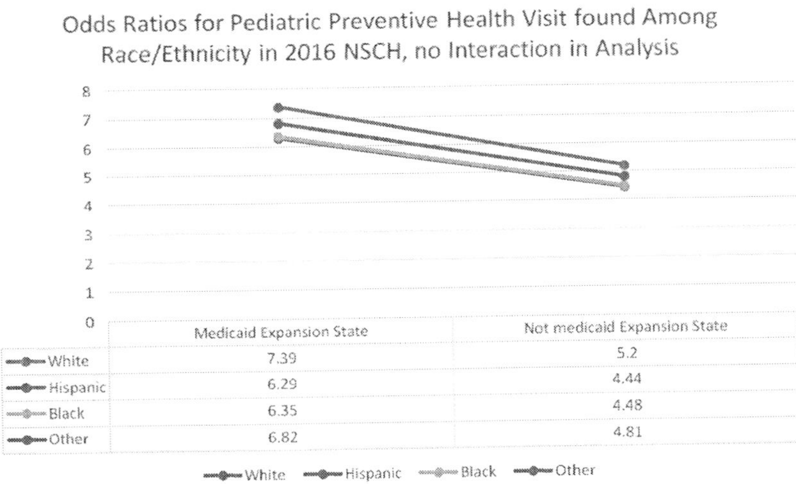

Figure 4. Odds ratios produced from the model that did not include a cross-level interaction between race/ethnicity and Medicaid expansion.
In this chart the interaction term is not used in the model. Black and Hispanic have similar odds ratios, Hispanic is obscured by Black. Hispanic is statistically significantly different from White, but Black and other are not.

Figure 4 is a chart comparing odds ratios among the racial/ethnic groups ignoring the interactions between Medicaid and PMV. In this model the odds ratio for PMV among children in expansion states is 1.42 times the odds ratio for children in non-expansion states 95% CI= [1.17, 1.72]. In this chart the slopes between Medicaid expansion and non-expansion states are equal because the interaction term is missing. All four race/ethnic categories of children in Medicaid Expansion states had greater odds ratios for PMV than children in the same categories in non-expansion states.

Discussion

These findings suggest that children in Medicaid expansion states had a higher probability of receiving a PMV than children in non-Medicaid expansion states. The results from the models with and without interaction terms both suggest that Medicaid expansion potentially had a positive effect on children's receipt of PMV, regardless of race or ethnicity. The reduced log-odds for children who are Black or Hispanic echo findings of disparities in insurance coverage among racial/ethnic groups after passage of the ACA (14). Disparities among the races and ethnicities remain in both expansion and non-expansion states and appear to be amplified in expansion states. This finding, which seemed counter-intuitive, appears to fit a pattern of exaggerated disparities that occur when health systems undergo reform (29). The 2013 annual report from the Agency for Healthcare Research and Quality suggested that states with higher health care quality scores also tended to have higher disparities among racial and ethnic groups, while states with lower health care quality scores tended to show lower disparities in care among racial and ethnic groups (30, 31).

Historic and systemic inequities (for example, the Home Owners Loan Corporation's "redlining", or color-coding, of neighborhoods by race and associating lending risk with the color coding) removed vulnerable populations to less desirable and less served areas, making it harder to physically get to healthcare providers. Systemic inequity reduced vulnerable populations' ability to receive and understand information (for example, by 2014 sixteen states had passed laws regulating navigators—assistants who help vulnerable populations in understanding and purchasing insurance in the ACA marketplace (30, 32)) and created disparities in the ways that vulnerable populations were able to take advantage of healthcare reform. Although all groups in the expanded states are receiving PMV at higher rates than their corresponding groups in non-expanded states, our results suggest that White children seem better positioned to take advantage of the changes in healthcare.

PMVs are considered critical components of children's health and wellbeing, particularly in relationship to ongoing surveillance of physical and developmental health concerns. That children in Medicaid expansion states have an increased probability of receiving PMV resonates with the well-known impact that having affordable insurance can have on accessing healthcare. That said, while the expansion of ACA creates an opportunity for affordable healthcare, it does not completely relieve populations from the ongoing effects of other social determinants of healthcare access.

It is notable that disparities continue to exist in ACA expansion states, and potentially speaks to the greater realities of accessing healthcare for many minority families, particularly those experiencing poverty (10). The ACA makes health insurance more affordable for more families, but it does not alleviate all barriers to healthcare. Impoverished children's caregivers are more likely to have caretakers working multiple jobs in order to make ends meet and may have less flexible schedules available to coordinate healthcare visits. Furthermore, transportation concerns may be more frequent in minority populations who may have less reliable sources of transportation, forcing parents to cancel appointments because of transportation issues. Lack of transportation could be compounded by the fact that minority populations are also more likely to live in a "medical desert," an area where few or no health care providers are available (25). While the ACA has had beneficial effects, it is one policy aimed at eliminating disparities painted on a canvas of 150 years of policy that created disparities (30). Even as Medicaid expansion accentuated disparities in children's receipt of PMV it simultaneously reduced barriers to PMV and is helping break the cycle of disadvantaged populations who have carried a disproportionate burden of morbidity and mortality in the US.

Ultimately, the data presented here indicate that ACA expansion is associated with some degree of improvement in healthcare access for all children; however, being in an ACA expansion state does not necessarily ensure ready access for all. The issues of poverty, transportation, medical deserts, and other social maladies more likely to be faced by minority populations continue to exacerbate unequal healthcare access, even in ACA expanded states. To be sure, a key to open the door to a healthcare office is a good thing, but if there is no road to the door, or a reliable means of transportation, then some citizens will still not have access to affordable healthcare.

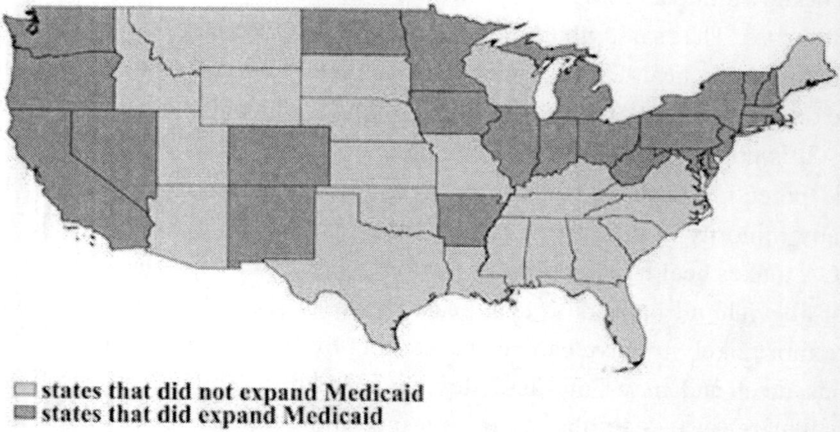

Figure 5. States that expanded Medicaid prior to data collection for the 2016 NSCH. This map illustrates the geographic clustering of states that did and did not expand Medicaid before 2016 NSCH data collection.

Limitations

The current analysis is largely framed as a consideration of healthcare access in relation to ACA expansion with an emphasis of ongoing racial and ethnic discrepancies in PMV receipt. The differences between receipt of PMV among the race/ethnic categories in this study might be attributable to other predictors not included in our models, including the demographics of the states. Perhaps differences in the racial/ethnic makeup, rurality, poverty, or other political policies of the states that expanded and did not expand may account for the differences we found. Another study might be strengthened by including state level variables that measure these differences. Prior research (27) suggests that there is spatial autocorrelation among the states that expanded and did not expand Medicaid. Figure 5 is a map of the states that expanded Medicaid in the time period before data collection for the 2016 NSCH illustrating their geographic clustering. The states that chose to expand Medicaid may share similar demographic and political characteristics, and the states that did not chose to expand may share different demographic and political characteristics. Another limitation is that the study is does not include individual level predictors that could account for health care consumption. The inclusion of such predictors might improve the model, but with a cost of increased multicollinearity and potential model misspecification.

Future work

The next step for this inquiry is to apply a similar analysis to the 2017 NSCH (4). Since Medicaid has continued to expand; the newer survey would include more states that have expanded and may paint a different picture of the impact of Medicaid expansion on pediatric PMV. It may also be informative to compare older versions of the NSCH from 2007 and 2012 to consider how these relationships have changed over time, though changes in the NSCH design will prevent firm comparison. Further investigation into differences in state policy regarding how providers interact with Medicaid would also provide beneficial information. Additionally, there may be subtle factors influencing the provider's willingness to accept Medicaid patients and that may have an impact on pediatric PMV.

REFERENCES

[1] Health Reform Tracker. Medicaid: changes under the ACA, 2018.

[2] Buettgens D. The cost of not expanding Medicaid: An updated analysis. Robert Wood Johnson Foundation. Urban Institute, 2017. URL: https://www.rwjf.org/en/library/research/2017/04/the-cost-of-not-expanding-medicaid.html.

[3] Hudson JL, Moriya AS. Medicaid expansion for adults had measurable 'welcome mat' effects on their children. Health Aff (Millwood) 2017;36(9):1643–51.

[4] Child and Adolescent Health Measurement Initiative (CAHMI), Data Resource Center for Child and Adolescent Health. 2016 National Survey of Children's Health: Child and Family Health Measures and Subgroups, SAS Codebook, Version 2.0, 2018.

[5] Hagan JF, Shaw JS, Duncan PM. Bright futures: guidelines for health supervision of infants, children, and adolescents, 3rd ed. Elk Grove Village, IL: American Academy of Pediatrics, 2017.

[6] Gunville J. The development of a prenatal care health literacy instrument for American Indian mothers. Int Public Health J 2019, in press.

[7] Walker C, Lui A. Power of the parents: Leveraging pediatric stakeholders to break the cycle of educational disparities. Int Public Health J 2019, in press.

[8] Quizhpi, C. Assessing the feasibility of integrating trauma-informed practices into primary pediatric care. Int Public Health J 2019, in press.

[9] Masiosek MV, Coffield AB, Flottemesch TE, Edwards NM, Solberg LI. Greater use of preventive services in U.S. health care could save lives at little or no cost. Health Affs (Millwood) 2010;20(9):1656-60.

[10] Flores, G. Racial and ethnic disparities in the health and health care of children. Pediatrics 2010;125(4):e979-e1020.

[11] Terui S. Conceptualizing the pathways and processes between language barriers and health disparities: review, synthesis, and extension. J Immigrant Minor Health 2017;19(1):215-24.

[12] Raphael JL, Guadagnolo BA, Beal AC, Giardino AP. Racial and ethnic disparities in indicators of a primary care medical home for children. Acad Pediatr 2009;9(4):221–7.

[13] Centers for Disease Control and Prevention. Preventive health care, gateway to health communication and social marketing practice, 2018. URL: https://www.cdc.gov/prevention/

[14] Artiga S, Orgera K. Changes in health coverage by race and ethnicity since implementation of the ACA, 2013-2017. Kaiser Family Foundation, 2019. URL: https://www.kff.org/disparities-policy/issuebrief/changes-in-health-coverage-by-race-and-ethnicity-since-implementation-of-the-aca-2013-2017.

[15] Bhatt CB, Beck-Sagué CM. Medicaid expansion and infant mortality in the United States. Am J Public Health 2018;108(4):565-7.

[16] Akande M, Minneci PC, Deans KJ, Xiang H, Chisolm DJ, Cooper JN. Healthcare delivery, quality, and safety: Effects of Medicaid expansion on disparities in trauma care and outcomes in young adults. J Surg Res 2018;228:42-5.

[17] Jenkins JM. Healthy and ready to learn: Effects of a school-based public health insurance outreach program for kindergarten-aged children. J School Health,2018;88(1):44-53.

[18] Graaf G, Snowden, L. Medicaid waivers and public sector mental health service penetration rates for youth. Am J Orthopsychiatry 2018;88(5):597–607.

[19] Remler DK, Korenman SD, Hyson RT. Estimating the effects of health insurance and other social programs on poverty under the Affordable Care Act. Health Affairs 2017;36 (10),1828-37.

[20] Venkataramani M, Pollack CE, Roberts ET. Spillover effects of adult Medicaid expansions on children's use of preventive services. Pediatrics 2017;140(6): e20170953.

[21] Andersen RM. Revisiting the behavioral model and access to medical care: Does it matter? J Health Soc Behav 1995;36(1):1-10.

[22] Yu SM, Bellamy HA, Kogan MD, Dunbar, JL, Schwalberg RH, Schuster MA. Factors that influence receipt of recommended preventive pediatric health and dental care. Pediatrics 2002;110(6):e73.

[23] Pylypchuk Y, Hudson J. Immigrants and the use of preventive care in the United States. Health Econ 2009;18(7):783–806.

[24] Yong AG, Lemyre L, Farrell SJ, Young MY. Acculturation in preventive health for immigrants: A systematic review on influenza vaccination programs in a socio-ecological framework. Canadian Psychol 2016;57(4):340.

[25] Medical deserts in America: Why we need to advocate for rural healthcare. URL: https://globalhealth.harvard.edu/blog/medical-deserts-america-why-we-need-advocate-rural-healthcare.

[26] National Council of State Legislatures. Affordable care act Medicaid expansion. URL: www.ncsl.org/research/health/ affordable-care-act-expansion.aspx,2018.

[27] Daniel P. Domain and time spatial analysis of Medicaid expansion and pediatric preventive health visit in pre-expansion and post-expansion states. Paper presented to Spatial Health Methods. Atlanta, GA, 2018 Dec 7.

[28] Raudenbush SW, Byrk,AS. Hierarchical linear models. Thousand Oaks, CA: Sage, 2019.

[29] Dawes DE. Presentation to Health Systems Symposium, Georgia Department of Public Health. Savannah, GA, 2019 May 13-14.

[30] Dawes DE, Satcher D. 150 years of ObamaCare, 1 ed. Baltimore, MD: Johns Hopkins University Press, 2016.

[31] National Healthcare Quality and Disparities Reports. URL: https://www.ahrq.gov/research/findings/nhqrdr/index.html.

[32] Navigator Regulation: Enacted Laws and Regulations. URL: https://www.naifa.org/advocacy/state-issues-positions-(2014-2017)/sinp/navigator-regulation-enacted-laws.

In: Child Environmental Health Disparities ISBN: 978-1-53617-823-4
Editors: IL Rubin and J Merrick

Chapter 11

SELF-PERCEIVED NEIGHBORHOOD QUALITY AND CHILDREN'S DEPRESSION SYMPTOMS IN A GENTRIFYING NORTHERN MANHATTAN

Teresa Durham[1], BS, Amy Margolis[1,2], PhD, David Pagliaccio[2], PhD, Wanda Garcia[1,5], MHA, Kylie Wheelock Riley[1], MPH, Jia Guo[1,4], MS, Shuang Wang[1,4], PhD, Bradley S Peterson[6], MD, Virginia Rauh[1,5], ScD and Julie B Herbstman[1,7,*], PhD

[1]Columbia Center for Children's Environmental Health, Columbia University Mailman School of Public Health,
[2]Division of Child and Adolescent Psychiatry and the Center for Developmental Neuropsychiatry, Department of Psychiatry, New York State Psychiatric Institute and the Columbia University College of Physicians and Surgeons, [3]Division of Clinical Developmental Neuroscience, Sackler Institute, New York State Psychiatric Institute, [4]Department of Biostatistics, Columbia University Mailman School of Public Health,
[5]Heilbrunn Department of Population & Family Health, Columbia University Mailman School of Public Health,

[*] Corresponding Author's Email: jh2678@cumc.columbia.edu.

[6]Institute for the Developing Mind, Children's Hospital Los Angeles and Keck School of Medicine, University of Southern California, Los Angeles, California and [7]Department of Environmental Health Sciences, Columbia University Mailman School of Public Health, New York, United States of America

Abstract

Poor neighborhood quality (NQ) is associated with social withdrawal and low self-esteem, as well as increased symptoms of anxiety and depression. The majority of reports assessing the association between NQ and child mental health use Census data, which rely on objective components of neighborhood composition and cannot capture a resident's perception of the neighborhood environment. This study used longitudinal measures of maternal self-reported NQ to assess the impact of NQ patterns in middle childhood on children's mental health, in a low-income, minority population that largely resides in gentrifying Northern Manhattan neighborhoods. When children were 5, 7, 9 and 11 years old, self-reported neighborhood information was collected, and neighborhood stress was used as the metric for NQ. Symptoms of anxiety and depression were assessed using the Revised Children's Manifest Anxiety Scale (RCMAS) and the Children's Depression Rating Scale (CDRS) in early adolescence at age 9-12 years. Children of mothers who rated their total NQ as "stressed" in middle childhood had significantly more symptoms of depression than children of mothers who reported their NQ as "non-stressed" ($p = 0.046$). Additionally, there was an observable difference in the number of individuals who reported clinically significant counts of depressive symptoms between mothers who reported stressed versus non-stressed NQ (10% vs. 6%, $p = 0.20$). There was, however, no association between NQ and total anxiety. Unlike Census data, self-report NQ assessments can be used as a tool to gauge residents' subjective experience in the neighborhood and to highlight how gentrification may benefit some child residents disproportionately.

Introduction

Over the past 20 years, the relationship between neighborhood composition and children's health has become increasingly well-established. Depending on the quality and frequency of a child's interactions with his or her neighborhood, environmental context can shape youth developmental outcomes. Variations in neighborhood quality (NQ) have been associated with childhood and adolescent cognitive differences in educational achievement, verbal ability, and working memory (1–8). With regard to socioemotional outcomes, stronger neighborhood economic resources, increased resident involvement, and increased resident employment are associated with better parent report of children's mental health and fewer parent-reported internalizing behaviors, such as social withdrawal and low self-esteem (9–11). Conversely, both living in a low socioeconomic status (SES) neighborhood and exposure to violence have been associated with increased levels of child and adolescent symptoms of depression and anxiety, as measured through parent and self-report (11–14).

In the field of children's health, this body of research emphasizes that investigations into environmental influences on children's mental development cannot be fully complete without considering the neighborhoods in which they live and grow. Despite robust NQ examinations, there remains a gap between analyses utilizing Census data and those that use residents' self-reported NQ assessments. Most studies observing a significant relationship between neighborhood makeup and children's health use area-level measures (e.g., Census), which rely on sociodemographic measurements of income, racial and ethnic composition, residential instability, and unemployment (15). While Census collections can be thorough, they are entirely objective, and some researchers argue they have the potential to weaken the observed linkage between place of residence and health (16). The systematically collected material does not measure neighborhood context and how individuals subjectively perceive their environment, in turn silencing elements of neighborhood satisfaction, structural and institutional problems in the neighborhood, relations with neighbors, and feelings of safety, all of which have been associated with resident well-being (17).

Furthermore, the use of Census data in children's environmental health studies is insufficient when trying to capture quickly changing neighborhood characteristics and how these might impact NQ perception and children's health, as a Census is only collected once every 10 years. This limitation, in addition to the Census' inability to capture an individual's perception of the neighborhood, is particularly relevant when monitoring how low-income, minority children are affected by the rapid gentrification of urban American cities. Importantly, this growing and often neglected demographic is more likely to live in disadvantaged, urban neighborhoods, due to the historical social and economic isolation of poor communities of color (1, 18–20). Many of such neighborhoods, including the neighborhood of participants in the present study, are quickly being gentrified (20, 21); however, how this phenomenon is impacting the health of existing child residents is largely unexplored.

Gentrification refers to the transformation of low-income, divested communities through the influx of investment and new residents with high SES (22, 23). Resulting increases in taxes and property value often raise the community's cost of living, creating a significant financial burden for long-time residents (24). While Census data can measure long-term socioeconomic differences in NQ following reinvestment, it cannot measure how some residents may benefit from gentrification dispropor-tionately and how this may influence perception of the neighborhood. This is an important distinction, as research suggests parent perception of NQ can act as a mediator between neighborhood environment and children's health (3, 25).

Thus, a gap in children's environmental health literature is evidenced by the shortage of analyses exploring the impact of longitudinal self-perceived NQ on children's mental health. This gap is especially relevant as researchers begin to analyze the health consequences of low-income, minority children residing in gentrifying communities. The goal of this study was to strengthen the relationship between longitudinal self-perceived NQ and differences in children's mental health (see Figure 1). We believe that after this relationship is established, future studies should connect individual NQ differences with indicators of neighborhood gentrification. Combined, this research can reveal the disproportionate benefits to children of reinvestment in a community and, ultimately, identify levers that can help all children living in gentrifying neighborhoods benefit from reinvestment, thereby breaking the cycle between self-perceived stressed NQ and children's mental health (see Figure 2).

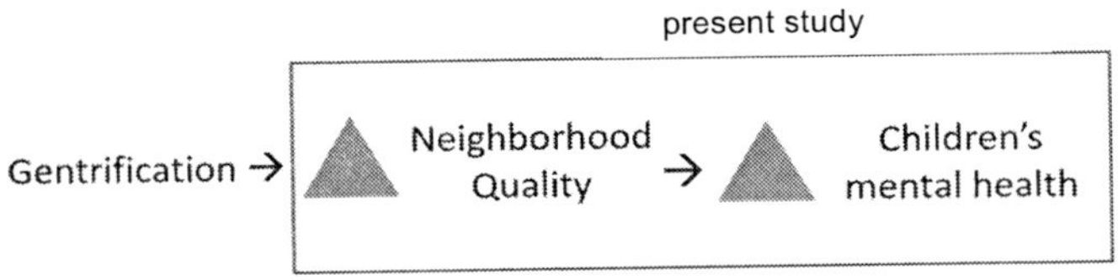

Figure 1. Conceptual framework for analysis of impacts of neighborhood quality on children's anxiety and depression symptoms.

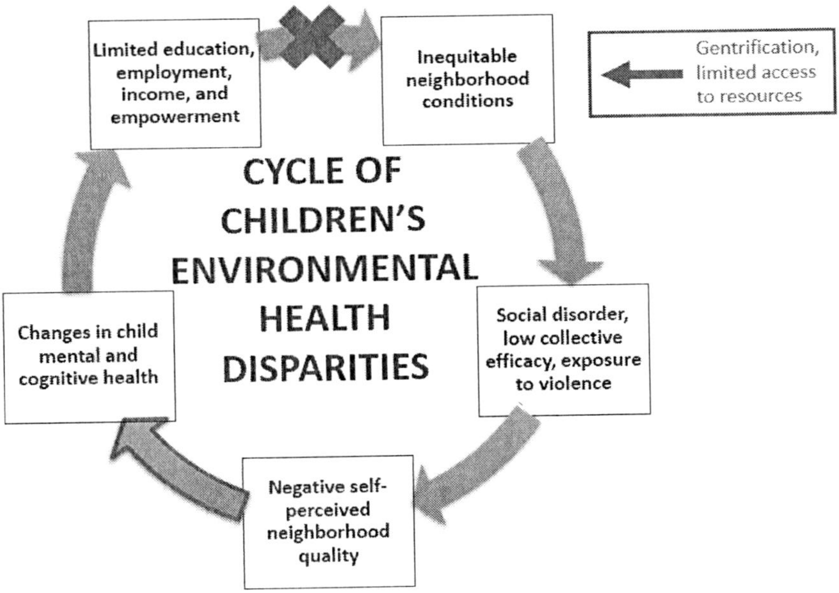

Figure 2. Breaking the cycle of environmental health disparities related to neighborhood quality and children's mental health.

Our Study

Study subjects were participants in the Mothers and Newborns Study, a prospective longitudinal birth cohort at the Columbia Center for Children's Environmental Health (CCCEH). Between 1998 and 2006, CCCEH recruited 727 women ages 18-35 years into the study from the prenatal clinics of New York Presbyterian Medical Center, Harlem Hospital, or their satellite clinics (26). Subjects were Dominican and African American women residing in Northern Manhattan (Washington Heights, Central Harlem) or the South Bronx. Enrollment exclusion criteria included smoking or use of other tobacco products during pregnancy, illicit drug use, first prenatal visit after 20th week of pregnancy, and the following pre-existing conditions: diabetes, hypertension, or known HIV infection. All study protocols were approved by the Institutional Review Board of Columbia University. Before each visit, mothers were informed about all study procedures and provided written informed consent to participate.

Neighborhood quality (NQ) assessment

When children were 5, 7, 9, and 11 years old, mothers were given a 32-question self-reported NQ assessment. The repeated administration of the questionnaire was intended to evaluate patterns of NQ over time across middle childhood. The questionnaire was adapted from existing measures of NQ (27–29), and consisted of three subscales, each used to assess different subjective aspects of neighborhood composition. Subscales included social order/disorder (12 questions), safety and violence (seven questions), and social cohesion and neighborhood stability (13 questions). Content in the social order/disorder and safety and violence subscales was rated based on level of agreement (0-4), while components of the social cohesion and neighborhood stability subscale were evaluated through yes/no responses. Examples from each include "Homeless/unemployed people are hanging around" (social order/disorder), worried about "Letting children go outside during the day/night" (safety and violence), and "My neighborhood is a good place to live" (social cohesion and neighborhood stability). The full questionnaire can be found in the Supplemental File.

Anxiety and depression assessments

Anxiety and depression symptoms were assessed once in early adolescence when children were between 9-12 years.

RCMAS – Revised Children's Manifest Anxiety Scale

The level and nature of anxiety symptoms in children were measured using the Revised Children's Manifest Anxiety Scale (RCMAS), a self-administered 37-item assessment completed by the child. RCMAS is divided into three subscales including physiological anxiety, worry and oversensitivity, and social concerns and concentration. Answering "yes" indicates that the item is descriptive of the child's feelings; higher scores on the assessment indicate increased levels of anxiety. Raw scores above 18 signal significant levels of anxiety that warrant further clinical assessment.

CDRS – Children's Depression Rating Scale

Level and severity of depressive symptoms were measured using the Children's Depression Rating Scale (CDRS) in a semi-structured interview administered by a trained research worker to the child. The CDRS includes 17 symptom areas encompassing cognitive, somatic, affective, and psychomotor symptoms. Examples include depressed feelings, difficulty having fun, depressed facial affect, and self-esteem. For 14 items, children rate on a 7-point scale, while the remaining three items are rated on a 5-point scale. Possible total scores range from 17-113. Any score above or equal to 40 signals significant levels of depression, whereas any score below or equal to 28 is often used to define minimal or no symptoms.

Statistical analysis

There were n = 727 mother and child pairs with available data on self-perceived NQ gathered at any one of the assessing time points: child ages 5, 7, 9, and 11 years. Of 727, 379 children had available data on anxiety symptoms measured through the RCMAS, and 372 children had available data on depression symptoms measured through the CDRS (see Figure 3).

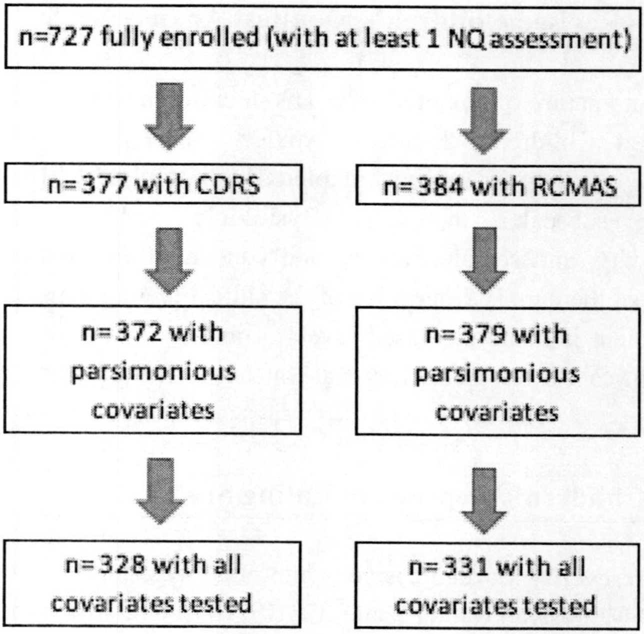

Figure 3. Flow Chart of Inclusion detailing how participants were selected for inclusion; parsimonious covariates include age at testing, sex, and ethnicity.

To analyze NQ, each participant's total NQ score and three individual subscale scores were standardized and scaled for the presence of stress. Items assessed through the 0-4 Likert scale were standardized such that all scores could be equally weighted and interpreted on a scale between 0-1 (0 = absence of stress, 1 = presence of stress). Subscale scores and total scores were found by taking the mean across all items. To analyze participants' patterns of NQ in middle childhood, group-based trajectory models using a latent class growth curve (LCGC) analysis were applied. Group-based trajectory models aim to identify clusters of individuals having similar NQ trajectories over the six-year period using finite mixture models (30). We modeled total and individual subscale scores, varying numbers of groups (1–4) and shapes (linear, quadratic, cubic). We selected the best fitting model for each NQ outcome (total NQ, social order/disorder, safety and violence, and social cohesion and neighborhood stability) using the

Bayesian Information Criterion (BIC), as well as the magnitude of group membership posterior probabilities. We evaluated change in BIC ($\Delta BIC \approx \log_e(B_{10})$) to compare increasingly complex models vs. the simpler (null) models and selected the final model based on the inflection point at which the ΔBIC leveled off (30, 31). These analyses were conducted using the SAS Proc TRAJ macro (31). Proc TRAJ will use any data provided to include the individual in the model that best fits them; individuals need not have all data points to be included.

To assess the association between patterns of NQ in middle childhood and symptoms of anxiety and depression in early adolescence, we examined eight multiple linear regression models, focusing on total NQ as our main exposure of interest. Prior to modeling, we assessed the distribution of RCMAS and CDRS to confirm that they were approximately normally distributed. NQ trajectory group was used as the independent variable, where separate models were fit to assess the association between total NQ, neighborhood social order/disorder, neighborhood safety and violence, and social cohesion and neighborhood stability and symptoms of anxiety (from RCMAS) and symptoms of depression (from CDRS) as the dependent variables. To isolate the effect of NQ on the presentation of anxiety and depression symptoms, we evaluated the inclusion of known or suspected risk factors for anxiety or depression symptoms based on the literature and our previous research (32). These included sex, age (in months) of child at testing, ethnicity, mother's intelligence (measured by the Test of Nonverbal Intelligence 3rd Edition, TONI-3) (33), maternal education (completion of high school prior to birth of this child vs. no completion), and maternal demoralization (measured by the Psychiatric Epidemiology Research Instrument–Demoralization (PERI-D) scale) (34). Final models included child sex, ethnicity, and age at testing, based on their statistically significant (at $p = 0.10$) association with either or both RCMAS and CDRS. Additionally, we explored stratified sex-specific associations between NQ and symptoms of anxiety and depression.

FINDINGS

A breakdown of participant characteristics is listed in Table 1. While there were no statistically significant differences among children included and excluded from this analysis, those included were slightly more likely to be female, African American, have lower maternal IQ and have mothers who were less likely to complete high school. At the time of enrollment, a majority of the participants resided in Northern Manhattan, a residential, non-tourist region of New York City that has been quickly gentrifying for the past 20 years (21, 35).

Table 1. Characteristics of subjects included (n = 386) and excluded (n = 342) from this analysis among 727 fully enrolled participants

Characteristic	Included in final model for CDRS or RCMAS (n = 386)	Excluded from final models (n = 342)	p-value
Sex (Female)	209 (54.1%)	167 (49.0%)	0.16
Race (African American)	146 (37.8%)	108 (31.7%)	0.08
Maternal Education (Completed High School)	233 (61.5%)	223 (66.8%)	0.14
Maternal TONI score[1]	20.0 (SD 8.6)	21.4 (8.8)	0.07
Maternal demoralization score[1,2]	1.16 (SD 0.64)	1.14 (SD 0.62)	0.68

[1] mean ± SD

[2] Range of demoralization: 0-3.3, where higher scores indicate more demoralization.

After total and subscale NQ data were standardized and scaled for the presence of stress, the best fitting group-based trajectory model yielded a binary separation of maternal self-reported NQ over the six-year assessment period in middle childhood. This result is shown in Table 2, where, for all four NQ outcomes, the two-group model showed the greatest change in BIC when comparing between models with different number of trajectory groups. Thus, NQ results suggested two distinct groups of NQ patterns across middle childhood, namely persistently "stressed" over time and persistently "non-stressed" over time. Participant characteristics by total NQ group assignment are presented in Table 1. It is noteworthy that mothers who were categorized as living in more stressed neighborhoods are less likely to have completed high school (p = 0.02), have a lower TONI score (p = 0.003) and have more demoralization (p = 0.009) than participants in the non-stressed neighborhoods. Raw individual trajectories for total NQ are shown in Figure 4A, while mean total NQ values at each time point are presented in Figure 4B. Figure 4B also shows percent breakdown of the two groups, with 41% of mothers (n = 158) persistently rating their total neighborhood composition as stressed, and 59% of mothers (n = 228) rating their neighborhood as being non-stressed. While all subscales were correlated, the trajectory pattern of the neighborhood safety and violence subscale was most similar to that of overall NQ (see Figure 5).

Table 2. BIC and BIC change between different number of NQ trajectory groups

Number of Groups	BIC	Null Model	ΔBIC*
NQ (total)			
1	470.19		
2	**726.79**	**1**	**256.6**
3	768.84	2	42.05
4	787.28	3	18.44
NQ (social order/disorder)			
1	153.12		
2	**369.11**	**1**	**215.99**
3	421.81	2	52.7
4	429.92	3	8.11
NQ (safety and violence)			
1	-175.84		
2	**21.83**	**1**	**197.67**
3	32.93	2	11.1
4	44.76	3	11.83
NQ (social cohesion & neighborhood stability)			
1	-642.46		
2	**-512.8**	**1**	**129.66**
3	-485.84	2	26.96
4	-484.46	3	1.38

*BIC = Bayesian Information Criterion.

*ΔBIC: BIC change between a more complex model and null model.

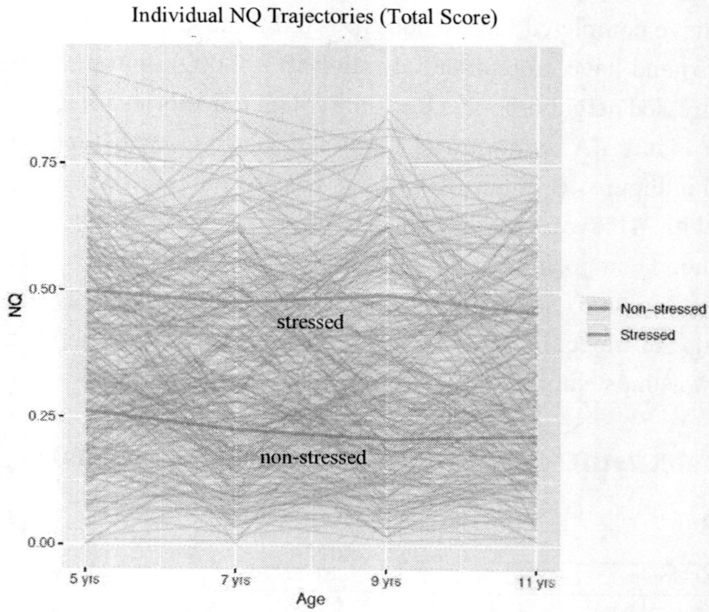

Figure 4A. All individual total NQ trajectories across middle childhood revealing distinct separation between stressed and non-stressed trajectory groups.

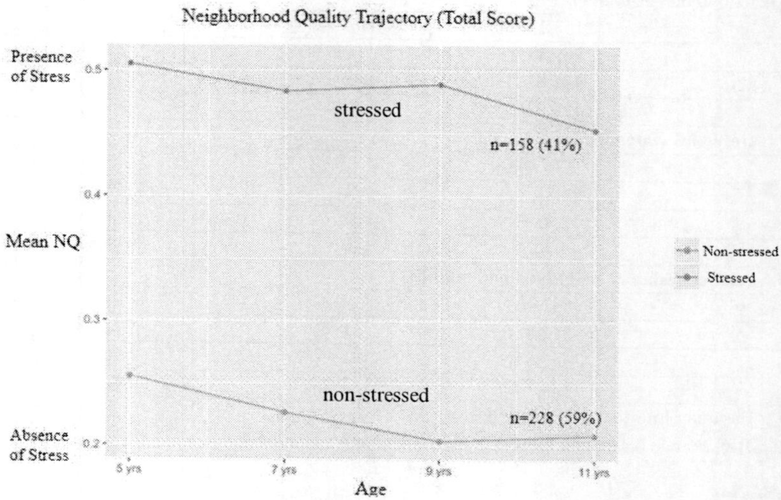

Figure 4B. Total NQ trajectory grouping by mean showing percent breakdown between stressed and non-stressed trajectory groups.

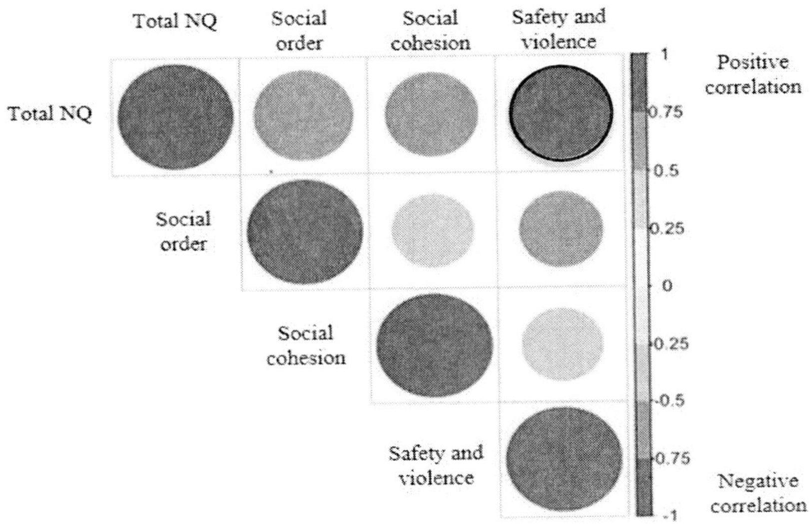

Figure 5. Correlations between total and subscale neighborhood quality trajectories showing strongest correlation between total NQ and safety and violence subscale.

Table 3. Association between NQ trajectories (stressed vs. non-stressed) and anxiety and depression symptoms measured by the CDRS and RCMAS

	CDRS (beta, 95% CI)		RCMAS (beta, 95% CI)	
	Univariate	**Adjusted***	**Univariate**	**Adjusted***
N	372	372	379	379
Stressed NQ	1.53 (0.004, 3.06)	1.56 (0.03, 3.08)	0.09 (-1.14, 1.32)	0.13 (-1.10, 1.36)
Not stressed NQ	ref	ref	ref	ref
Age at assessment	-0.14 (-0.78, 0.51)	-0.08 (-0.72, 0.56)	-0.87 (-1.39, -0.35)	-0.86 (-1.38, -0.34)
Dominican	--	-0.78 (-1.55, -0.001)	--	-0.39 (-1.01, 0.24)
African American	--	ref	--	ref
Female	--	-0.23 (-1.73, 1.28)	--	-0.75 (-1.96, 0.47)
Male	--	ref	--	ref

* Adjusted models include sex, child age at testing and ethnicity.

We found that stressed NQ across middle childhood was not associated with any observable difference in anxiety symptoms in early adolescence (see Table 3). However, persistently stressed NQ was associated with higher levels of depression symptoms in this age group (see Table 3). After controlling for sex, ethnicity, and child age at testing, Figure 6 shows that children of mothers in the stressed NQ trajectory group scored, on average, 1.5 points higher on the CDRS than those in the non-stressed trajectory group—and this difference was statistically significant with $p = 0.046$ ($\beta = 1.56$, 95% CI: 0.03, 3.08). Although not statistically significant, it is notable that more individuals obtained CDRS scores greater than 40 (clinical cutoff) in the stressed versus non-stressed NQ trajectory group (10% vs. 6%, $p = 0.20$; Figure 6). None of the three NQ subscale trajectories were individually predictive of children's depression scores (data not shown), and we found no significant sex-specific associations between NQ and either anxiety or depression symptoms (data not shown).

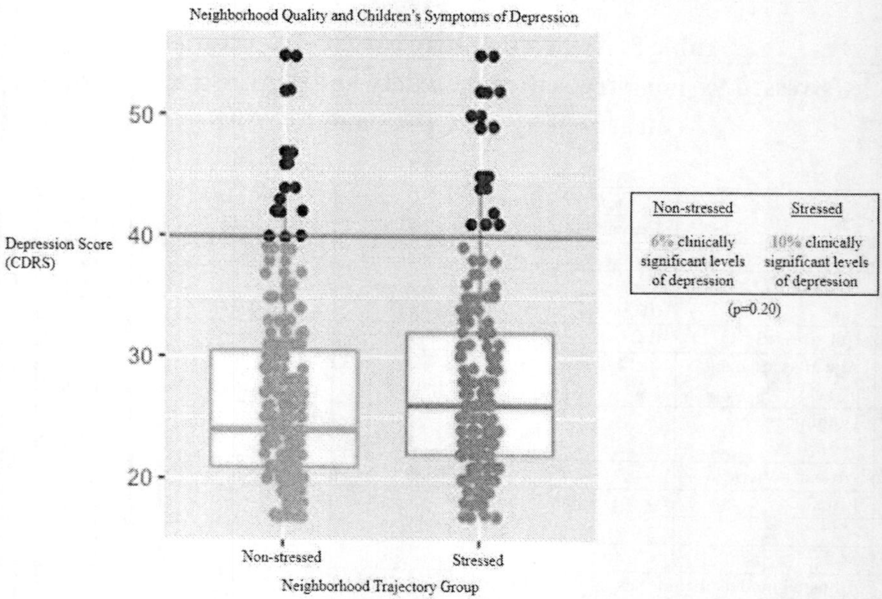

* red line marks cutoff for clinically significant levels of depression.

Figure 6. Difference in child report of depression symptoms between self-perceived stressed and non-stressed NQ as reported by mother.

DISCUSSION

In this study, we examined the association between longitudinal maternal self-reported NQ and children's self-report of symptoms of anxiety and depression. After controlling for other factors which may influence report of children's levels of symptoms of anxiety or depression, we observed that as mothers reported increasing levels of neighborhood stress, children reported increasing levels of symptoms of depression. Interestingly, while a number of sociodemographic factors were associated with NQ trajectory (e.g., education, IQ, demoralization), these were not significant predictors of child's report of depressive symptoms while self-perceived NQ trajectory was. Thus, maternal assessment of NQ may be an important predictor of childhood depression symptoms. Although we did not formally perform statistical tests of mediation, our findings support existing literature which suggests parent perception of NQ may act as a mediator between neighborhood environment and changes in children's mental health.

This research is relevant for the health and success of children living in stressed neighborhood environments. Depressive symptoms in childhood have been inversely associated with a child's ability to build social relationships, concentrate academically, and be self-reliant (36–38). Understanding the environmental factors that drive children's symptoms of depression, including those related to NQ, is important as researchers continue to direct effort towards breaking the cycle of children's mental illness, particularly for those low-income and minority children who are more likely to live in disadvantaged neighborhood environments and more susceptible to poor mental health (see Figure 2). In order for such efforts to be best targeted, researchers must be able to acquire the most informative measurement of NQ as a predictor of children's mental health. The growing body of research proposing neighborhoods as a source inequality relies heavily on SES and its association with children's development (3). Given the weaknesses inherent to Census collection data, these analyses might overlook important influences of neighborhood environment on children's health.

Rather than measuring objective neighborhood characteristics through Census, the self-reported NQ evaluation allows researchers to gauge neighborhood context and record how residents subjectively experience their surrounding environment. This is a useful tool considering that outside observation and resident perception of environmental stressors may not always converge (17). Furthermore, the repeated, longitudinal administration of the self-report assessment allows researchers to capture the effect of quickly changing neighborhood characteristics on perception of NQ, which contrasts most NQ research based on neighborhood residence at a single point in time (12). Thus, a subjective, long-term NQ assessment is more descriptive of the mechanisms through which a disadvantaged neighborhood environment may be linked to decreased mental health, and also better illustrates the mental, physical, and social dimensions that are known to shape a child's wellbeing (39).

These strengths of the self-report are particularly relevant as researchers analyze how gentrification impacts the health of existing low-income minority youth living in the neighborhood. This demographic is not only more likely to live in socially and economically under-resourced urban neighborhoods, it may also be more vulnerable to inequitable neighborhood conditions due to ongoing transformation of urban communities (40, 41). While direct effects of gentrification were not measured in this study, gentrification and its community health implications are interlaced in the context of our analysis. The children in this study live in Northern Manhattan, a neighborhood of New York City that has experienced rapid reinvestment. However, not all individuals residing in gentrifying neighborhoods, similar to this one, benefit from incoming resources. Using Census material to measure the benefits of reinvestment in a community may lead to the conclusion that gentrification is net positive for new and existing residents, as the data could reveal increases in median income and neighborhood diversity. Despite such socioeconomic changes, perceived neighborhood quality can remain constant for residents without access to the neighborhood's new amenities (e.g., upscale restaurants, commercial shopping districts), and also for residents displaced due to cost of living increase. In order to evaluate how certain children may benefit from gentrification disproportionately, a longitudinal, self-perceived NQ assessment is necessary. In future research, it may also be important to consider the role of large-scale public housing near or adjacent to gentrifying neighborhoods.

Study limitations

There are a number of noteworthy limitations to this analysis, mainly related to our inability to control for all possible stressors that may contribute to a child's presentation of anxiety and depression symptoms, leading to residual confounding. While the children included in this analysis were not statistically different than those who were excluded due to missing data, there were slight differences that might have influenced the results (see Table 1). Additionally, some researchers have suggested differential effects on child behavior from two-parent and single-parent households (25), which leads us to believe that variances in family structure may also have affected children's symptoms of depression. Previous research conducted among this same cohort has shown that housing instability, as defined by more than three residential moves in a seven year time frame, is related to behavioral differences in childhood (42). This provides an additional route for variance in children's mental development, one that can potentially be connected with gentrification and residential displacement in the future. Lastly, we recognize that we tested the effects of difference in NQ against two discrete endpoints—anxiety symptoms and depression symptoms. We did not adjust for multiple comparisons because there is independent literature suggesting investi-gation into both domains. Had we adjusted for multiple comparisons, our findings would not reach statistical significance with $p = 0.05$ due to the small sample size. Should researchers interpret this study as an exploratory, combined analysis between NQ and anxiety and depression symptoms, an adjustment for multiple comparisons would be necessary.

CONCLUSION

Through this study, we have shown that a mother's longitudinal assessment of her NQ is associated with her child's self-reported symptoms of depression in early adolescence. To more closely connect gentrification to children's mental health outcomes, future research should connect gentrification indicators and precise resident location directly with changes in self-reported NQ. Through this linkage, researchers can document the disproportionate impacts to children that reinvestment can bring to urban communities. Furthermore, this information can be used to identify levers that can be used to develop health-based policy interventions designed to help all children living in gentrifying neighborhoods benefit from reinvestment.

REFERENCES

[1] Ceballo R, McLoyd VC, Toyokawa T. The influence of neighborhood quality on adolescents' educational values and school effort. J Adolesc Res 2004;19(6):716–39.

[2] Munoz E, Scott S, Hyun J, Almeida D, Smith J, Sliwinski M. Perceived neighborhood quality and cognitive function: Contrasting effects en in-lab and ambulatory assessments. Gerontologist 2015;55(Suppl 2):825.

[3] Minh A, Muhajarine N, Janus M, Brownell M, Guhn M. A review of neighborhood effects and early child development: How, where, and for whom, do neighborhoods matter? Health Place 2017;46:155–74.

[4] Hicks AL, Handcock MS, Sastry N, Pebley AR. Sequential neighborhood effects: The effect of long-term exposure to concentrated disadvantage on children's reading and math test scores. Demography 2018;55(1):1–31.

[5] Garner CL, Raudenbush SW. Neighborhood effects on educational attainment?: A multilevel analysis. Sociol Educ 1991;64(4):251–62.

[6] Greenman E, Bodovski K, Reed K. Neighborhood characteristics, parental practices and children's math achievement in elementary school. Soc Sci Res 2011;40(5):1434–44.

[7] Benson J, Borman G. Family, neighborhood, and school settings across seasons: When do socioeconomic context and racial composition matter for the reading achievement growth of. Teach Coll Rec 2010;112(5):1338–90.

[8] Barajas RG, Philipsen N, Brooks-Gunn J. Cognitive and emotional outcomes for children in poverty. Handb Fam Poverty 2008;5:311–33.

[9] Xue Y, Leventhal T, Brooks-Gunn J, Earls FJ. Neighborhood residence and mental health problems of 5- to 11-year-olds. Arch Gen Psychiatry 2005;62(5):554–63.

[10] O'Campo P, Caughy MO, Nettles SM. Partner abuse or violence, parenting and neighborhood influences on children's behavioral problems. Soc Sci Med 2010;70(9):1404–15.

[11] Chen JJ, Brooks-Gunn J. Neighborhoods, schools, and achievement. In: Harris KR, Graham S, Urdan T, Graham S, Royer JM, Zeidner M, eds. APA Educ Psychol handbook: Individual differences and cultural and contextual factors, vol 2. Washington, DC: American Psychological association, 2011:337–60.

[12] Leventhal T, Brooks-Gunn J. Children in neighborhood contexts. Am Psychol Soc 2003;12(1):27–31.

[13] Aneshensel CS, Sucoff CA. The neighborhood context of adolescent mental health. J Health Soc Behav 1996;37(4):293–310.

[14] Leventhal T, Brooks-Gunn J. The neighborhoods they live in: The effects of neighborhood residence on child and adolescent outcomes. Psychol Bull 2000;126(2):309–37.

[15] Kohen DE, Brooks-Gunn J, Leventhal T, Hertzman C. Neighborhood income and physical and social disorder in Canada: Associations with young children's competencies. Child Dev 2002;73(6):1844–60.

[16] Wen M, Hawkley LC, Cacioppo JT. Objective and perceived neighborhood environment, individual SES and psychosocial factors, and self-rated health: An analysis of older adults in Cook County, Illinois. Soc Sci Med 2006;63(10):2575–90.

[17] Schaefer-McDaniel N. Neighborhood stressors, perceived neighborhood quality, and child mental health in New York City. Health Place 2009;15(1):148–55.

[18] William Julius Wilson. The truly disadvantaged: The inner city, the underclass and public policy. Chicago, IL: University of Chicago Press, 1987.

[19] Leventhal T, Fauth RC, Brooks-Gunn J. Neighborhood poverty and public policy: A 5-year follow-up of children's educational outcomes in the New York City moving to opportunity demonstration. Dev Psychol 2005;41(6):933–52.

[20] Thorpe R. Urban divestment, rural decline and the politics of mass incarceration. Good Soc 2014;23(1):17.

[21] Bergad L. Washington Heights/Inwood demographic, economic, and social transformations 1990-2005 with a special focus on the Dominican Population. New York: CUNY, 2008.

[22] Hackman DA, Betancourt LM, Gallop R, Romer D, Brodsky NL, Hurt H, et al. Mapping the trajectory of socioeconomic disparity in working memory: Parental and neighborhood factors. Child Dev 2014;85(4):1433–45.

[23] Davidson M, Lees L. New-build "gentrification" and London's riverside renaissance. Environ Plan A 2005;37(7):1165–90.

[24] Pearsall H. Moving out or moving in? Resilience to environmental gentrification in New York City. Local Environ 2012;17(9):1013–26.

[25] Shumow L, Vandell DL, Ponser J. Perceptions of danger: A psychological mediator of neighborhood demographic characteristics. Am J Orthopsychiatry 1998;68(3):468–78.

[26] Whyatt RM, Camann DE, Kinney PL, Reyes A, Ramirez J, Dietrich J, et al. Residential pesticide use during pregnancy among a cohort of urban minority women. Environ Health Perspec. 2002;110(5):507–14.

[27] Kim SY, Nair R, Knight GP, Roosa MW, Updegraff KA. Measurement equivalence of neighborhood quality measures for European American and Mexican American families. J Commun Psychol 2008;37(1):1–20.

[28] Samson R, Raudenbush S, Earls F. Neighborhoods and violent crime: A multilevel study of what influences collective efficacy. Word J Int Linguist Assoc 1997;277(8):918–24.

[29] Sampson RJ, Raudenbush SW. Systematic social observation of public spaces: A new look at disorder in urban neighborhoods. Am J Sociol 1999;105(3):603–51.

[30] Nagin DS. Group-based trajectory modeling: An overview. Ann Nutr Metab 2014;65:205–10.

[31] Jones B, Nagin D, Roeder K. A SAS procedure based on mixture models for estimating developmental trajectories. Sociol Methods Res 2001;29(3):374–93.

[32] Perera F, Nolte ELR, Wang Y, Margolis AE, Calafat A, Wang S, et al. Bisphenol A exposure and symptoms of anxiety and depression among inner city children at 10–12 years of age. Environ Res 2016;(151):195–202.

[33] Brown L, Sherbenou RJ, Johnsen SK. Test of nonverbal intelligence. J Psychoeduc Assess 2011;29(5):484–8.

[34] Dohrenwend BS, Askenasy AR, Krasnoff L, Dohrenwend BP. Exemplification of a method for scaling life events: The PERI Life Events Scale. J Health Soc Behav 1978;19(2):205–29.

[35] Wyly EK, Newman K. The right to stay put, revisited: Gentrification and resistance to displacement in New York city. Urban Stud 2006;43(1):23–57.

[36] Terrell L. Strayhorn. When race and gender collide: Social and cultural capital's influence on the academic achievement of African American and Latino males. Rev High Educ 2010;33(3):307–32.

[37] Fröjd SA, Nissinen ES, Pelkonen MUI, Marttunen MJ, Koivisto AM, Kaltiala-Heino R. Depression and school performance in middle adolescent boys and girls. J Adolesc 2008;31(4):485–98.

[38] Sacco WP, Graves DJ. Childhood depression, interpersonal problem-solving, and self-ratings of performance. J Clin Child Psychol 1984;13(1):10–5.

[39] Hill TD, Ross CE, Angel RJ. Neighborhood disorder, psychophysiological distress, and health. J Health Soc Behav 2005;46:170–86.

[40] Hill TD, Maimon D. Neighborhood context and mental health. In: Aneshensel CS, Phelan JC, Bierman A, eds. Handbook of the sociology of mental health. New York: Springer, 2002:479–501.

[41] Massey DS, Eggers ML. The ecology of inequality: Minorities and the concentration of poverty, 1970-1980. Am J Sociol 2002;95(5):1153–88.

[42] Gaylord AL, Cowell WJ, Hoepner LA, Perera FP, Rauh VA, Herbstman JB. Impact of housing instability on child behavior at age 7 years. Int Public Health J 2018;10(4):287–95.

In: Child Environmental Health Disparities ISBN: 978-1-53617-823-4
Editors: IL Rubin and J Merrick

Chapter 12

Water Infrastructure and Childhood Blood Lead Levels: Characterizing the Effects of Exclusion from Municipal Services in Wake County (NC, USA)

Allison C Clonch[1], MCRP, MSPH,
Michael Fisher[1], PhD
and Jacqueline MacDonald Gibson[1,2], PhD
[1]Department of Environmental Sciences and Engineering, Gillings School of Global Public Health, University of North Carolina, Chapel Hill, North Carolina and [2]Department of Environmental and Occupational Health, Indiana University, Bloomington, Indiana, United States of America

Abstract

Childhood lead exposure is associated with impaired cognitive development, decreased IQ levels, and increased rates of juvenile delinquency. Lack of access to municipal water services, which in some communities disproportionately affects Black neighborhoods, is associated with higher levels of lead in drinking water. Objectives: This study aims to characterize the effects of exclusion from municipal water infrastructure on childhood blood lead levels. Methods: We created a novel 16-year database of 34,314 children, with which we examined the effects of municipal water access on childhood blood lead levels in Wake County, NC. Using childhood blood lead data from 2002 to 2017, we used ordinary-least squares and logistic regression models with childhood blood lead levels as the primary outcome of interest and municipal water access at time of birth as the primary exposure of interest. Results: Our results suggest that a lack of access to municipal water is significantly associated with elevated blood lead levels. Children without municipal water service at birth had blood lead concentrations that were 0.12 µg/dL higher than children with municipal water. Children with access to municipal water service had significantly lower odds of having blood lead above the 'level of concern' as defined by the Centers for Disease Control than children with municipal water service (OR = 0.82). Conclusion: These findings support the need for more regulatory oversight and water quality tests of private water systems or facilitating access to municipal supplies in order to mitigate the impacts associated with childhood lead exposure.

INTRODUCTION

Approximately 535,000 children ages 1 to 5 years in the United States had a blood lead level above 5 µg/dL in 2018 (1). There is no safe concentration of blood lead in children, and lead exposure in childhood has long been known to impair intellectual and behavioral development (2). Young children are particularly susceptible to lead toxicity. Infants absorb 4 to 5 times more lead than older children and adults, and early childhood is a critical period of vulnerability to lead toxicity (3).

A lack of access to municipal water services is associated with elevated levels of lead in drinking water (4), especially among low-income and African-American neighborhoods (5). "Municipal underbounding" is the phenomenon whereby communities of color living adjacent to majority white municipalities are systematically excluded from incorporation (6–9). In the state of North Carolina, individuals outside of municipal service areas live in areas called extraterritorial jurisdictions (ETJs), and many of these households rely on private wells for water (10, 11). It has been demonstrated that land use planning and policy, at least in some jurisdictions, has discriminatorily excluded low-income and minority neighborhoods from municipal boundaries (6, 8, 9, 12–14). It has also been shown that race significantly predicts whether a community within an extraterritorial jurisdiction has municipal water services in North Carolina and Wake County, with predominantly Black neighborhoods being the least likely to have municipal water access (10, 11). The Safe Drinking Water Act in the United States sets an action level for lead in drinking water at 15 µg/L. However, the Safe Drinking Water Act only applies to community water systems, which are defined as those serving at least 15 service connections or 25 people year-round (15). Private wells, which are not protected by the Safe Drinking Water Act, are often overlooked as a source of lead exposure (4, 16).

The purpose of this project is to quantify the relationship between a lack of access to municipal water and childhood blood lead levels in Wake County, North Carolina, USA.

OUR STUDY

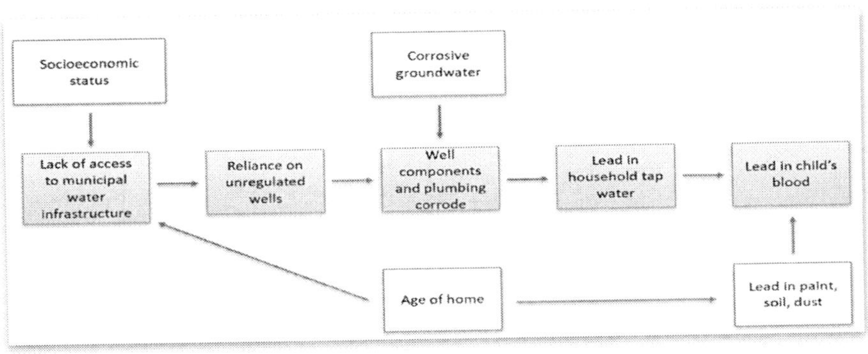

Figure 2. Conceptual model detailing the causal pathway between lack of access to municipal water and a child's observed blood lead with key covariates which may also affect either water access or lead exposure, such as socioeconomic status or age of the home.

We created a database of 34,314 observations at the level of the individual child spanning from 2002 to 2017 with data including children's blood lead, water access, location within an ETJ, demographic data, and other variables. Using this database, we used statistical models to estimate the effect of exclusion from municipal water services on childhood blood lead levels. Figure 1 illustrates the conceptual model used to create our statistical models.

Database development

Our retrospective database included tax parcel data from Wake County GIS Services, childhood blood lead data from North Carolina's Childhood Lead Poisoning Prevention Program (NC LEAD), and 2010 census data and 2017 American Community Survey (ACS) 5-year estimates data. NC LEAD provided all blood lead test results for children screened in Wake County between 2002 and 2017. The NC LEAD program requires health care providers across the state to report results of children's blood lead tests for surveillance purposes. While health care providers are encouraged to test blood lead for all children between the ages of 12 and 24 months, screening is mandatory for children enrolled in federal and state assistance programs (women, infants, and children; Medicaid; or Health Choice). The tax parcel data included in this study were for all residential parcels in Wake County from 2002 to 2018. All data cleaning and analysis was completed in STATA 15.1 (Statacorp, College Station, TX).

Merging all the yearly tax parcel files was the first step of creating the database. After acquiring the data, which is publicly available, we merged the yearly datasets using the unique PIN ID assigned to each parcel. If a parcel existed in multiple years of data, we kept the data for the first occurrence of the parcel, while incorporating all new parcel information that appeared in later years. Additionally, utility status and extraterritorial jurisdiction status were captured for each individual year for each parcel to determine when or if a parcel received municipal water access or if a parcel was incorporated into municipal boundaries. Utility data from Wake County

GIS services, which indicated municipal water access, were only reported from 2002-2010. To capture data timepoints after this, we supplemented our data set with tax parcel data from Wake County's revenue services department from 2013 and 2018; additional years of data were not available. Therefore, municipal water access data were incorporated from 2002-2010, 2013, and 2018. After this, all non-residential parcels were dropped from the dataset, leaving only parcels identified as dwellings.

Next, childhood blood lead data from the NC LEAD database were merged with the tax parcel data using the addresses from both datasets. The addresses were disaggregated into their parts (i.e., street name and number, city, zip) and cleaned for any possible variations between the two datasets (for example, RD versus road). We used an exact match on the datasets based on addresses, then STATA's DTALink function, which uses probabilistic linkage methods to score each potential pair of records on the probability the two records match, so that pairs with higher overall scores indicate a better match than pairs with lower scores. The merge parameters were iteratively revised and results reviewed until the parameters yielded results that included only exact matches and plausible inexact matches as determined from inspection of subsets of 100 matched entries.

Geocoding and spatial join

We used ArcMap (Version 10.6, ESRI, Redlands, CA) to geocode the data and perform a spatial join in order to merge ACS data to each observation. We geocoded the data in ArcMap using a stand-alone geocoding program created from ESRI's StreetMap Premium data for the year 2017 (StreetMap™ Premium for ArcGIS, ESRI, Redlands, CA). Fewer than 1% of the addresses were not matched; these were dropped from the dataset. We downloaded population demographics from the 2010 census and income data from the 2017 ACS 5-year estimates. We used a shapefile of Wake County to perform a spatial join to assign each observation from our dataset to a census block along with the corresponding census and ACS data.

Statistical models

For the analysis of the database, the primary outcome of interest was childhood blood lead concentration, and the primary exposure of interest was municipal water access at time of birth. We built an ordinary least squares regression model and two logistic regression models using blood lead benchmarks of 5 μg/dL and 2 μg/dL. For all models, we controlled for age in intervals of 18 months, gender, municipal status at time of birth, year of blood draw, home value in logarithmic form, year the home was built, median household income at the census block group, percent Black population at the census block, and percent Hispanic population at the census block.

FINDINGS

A total of 34,314 children from Wake County, NC, were included in the analyses. The mean blood lead level for the population was 1.7 μg/dL, and the mean age of the child at time of testing was 550 days (see Table 1). Males and females were evenly represented at 51% and 49% of the study population, respectively. Approximately 5.5% of individuals in the study population lived in extraterritorial jurisdictions, and 14.7% of individuals did not have municipal water access at time of birth (see Table 2).

Table 1. Summary statistics for key continuous variables included in the models.

Variables	Mean	Min	Max
Lead	1.65	1	35
Black, Percent	0.25	0.0022	0.93
Hispanic, Percent	0.1	0.0056	0.69
Year Tested		2002	2017
Year Built		1803	2017
Median Household Income	78600	17900	210000
Home Value (Log)	12.2	9.91	16.9
Age (Days)	550	0	2190

Table 2. Brief summary of dichotomous variables from the model. Summary statistics for key binomial variables included in the models

Variables		N	%
Water			
	Y	29,279	85.3
	N	5,035	14.7
ETJ			
	Y	1,871	5.5
	N	32,443	94.5
Gender			
	F	16,827	49
	M	17,487	51

Variables influencing blood lead levels in the study population

Access to municipal water and Black race were associated with children's blood lead levels (see Table 3). Children without municipal water service at birth had blood lead concentrations that were 0.12 µg/dL higher than children with municipal water. Blood lead levels increased, on average, by 0.023 µg/dL, for every 10% increase in the Black population proportion in the child's census block. In contrast, Hispanic population was not associated with blood lead levels. Year the child was tested was highly significant ($p < 0.0001$), with each additional year of time being associated with a decrease in blood lead levels of -0.092 µg/dL.

Similarly, the age of the child being between 18 to 36 months was highly significantly associated with an average increase in blood lead of 0.13 µg/dL from the referent (less than 18 months, $p < 0.0001$), and the age of the child being between 36 to 54 months was also significantly associated with an average increase in blood lead of 0.095 µg/dL ($p < 0.05$). Year the house was built was also highly significant at all levels when compared to the referent (built before 1950), with houses built between 2000 and 2005 being associated with the lowest level, a decrease of 0.55 µg/dL blood lead ($p < 0.0001$). Finally, home value in logarithmic form was highly significantly associated with a decrease of 0.22 µg/dL in blood lead level on average for every log-10 increase in home value ($p < 0.0001$). Thus, a two-fold increase in home value is associated with a decrease in blood lead levels of -0.066 µg/dL.

Table 3. Results of ordinary least squares regression model using blood lead levels as primary endpoint.

		R^2 = 0.1053
Variables	B	p-value
Water Access at Birth	-0.12	<0.0001
Year Tested	-0.092	<0.0001
Black Population fraction	0.23	<0.0001
Home Value (Log)	-0.22	<0.0001
Gender	0.037	0.0059
Municipal Status	0.038	0.24
Hispanic Population, percent	-0.085	0.44
Median Household Income	<0.0001	0.6
Age		
18 to 36 Months	0.13	<0.0001
36 to 54 Months	0.095	0.01
Over 54 Months	0.053	0.73
Year Household Built		
1970 to 1950	-0.33	<0.0001
1970 to 1990	-0.41	<0.0001
1990 to 2000	-0.5	<0.0001
2000 to 2005	-0.55	<0.0001
After 2005	-0.44	<0.0001
N	34314	

Variables influencing the odds of elevated blood lead levels in the study population

Children with access to municipal water service had significantly lower odds of having elevated blood lead above the 'level of concern' as defined by the Centers for Disease Control than children with municipal water service (see Table 4, Figure 2: OR = 0.82, $p < 0.05$). Similarly, these children had decreased odds of having blood lead concentrations above 2 µg/dL than children without water service (see Table 5, Figure 3: OR = 0.73, $p < 0.0001$). Year in which the child was tested was highly significantly associated with the odds of elevated blood lead levels when dichotomized at 5 μg/dL (see Table 4, Figure 2, OR = 0.81, $p < 0.0001$). The same effect was observed when blood lead was dichotomized at 2 μg/dL (see Table 5, Figure 3, OR = 0.78, $p < 0.0001$). Children living in census blocks with increasing fraction of Black population had significantly higher odds of elevated blood lead levels when dichotomized at 5 μg/dL (see Table 4, Figure 2, OR = 1.5, $p < 0.05$). Similarly, children living in census Blocks with increasing fraction of Black population had highly significantly increased odds of blood lead levels above 2 μg/dL (see Table 5, Figure 3, OR = 1.8, $p < 0.0001$).

Children living in census blocks with increasing percentage of Hispanic population did not have significantly increased odds of having elevated blood lead levels above 5 μg/dL (see Table 4, Figure 2, OR = 0.58, $p = 0.23$). However, when dichotomized at 2 μg/dL, children living in census blocks with an increasing fraction of Hispanic population did have significantly increased odds of having blood lead levels above 2 μg/dL (see Table 5, Figure 3: OR = 1.5, $p < 0.05$).

Table 4. Results of a logistic regression model of dichotomized blood lead level (above or below 5μg/dL).

	Pseudo R^2 = 0.0875	
Variables	**OR**	**p-value**
Water Access at Birth	0.82	0.021
Year Tested	0.81	<0.0001
Black Population Fraction	1.5	0.02
Hispanic Population Fraction	0.58	0.23
Home Value (Log)	0.65	<0.0001
Gender	1.1	0.26
Municipal Status	0.98	0.9
Median Household Income	1.0	0.9
Age		
18 to 36 Months	1.4	<0.0001
36 to 54 Months	1.3	0.01
Over 54 Months	2.8	0.17
Year Household Built		
1950 to 1970	0.48	<0.0001
1970 to 1990	0.43	<0.0001
1990 to 2000	0.33	<0.0001
2000 to 2005	0.29	<0.0001
After 2005	0.44	<0.0001
N	34314	

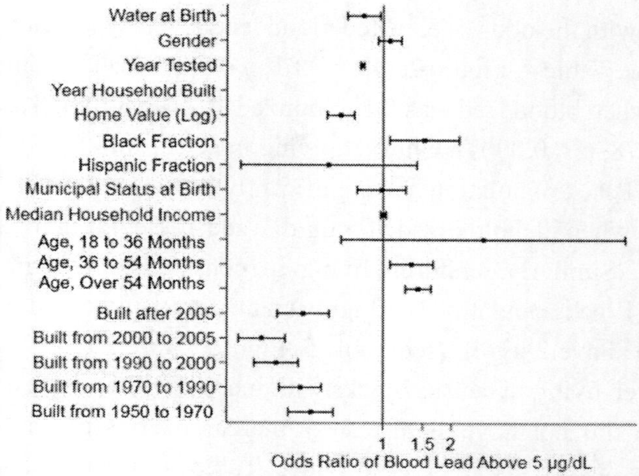

Figure 2. Graphical representation of the 5 µg/dL logistic model with odds ratios, confidence intervals, and all variables included in model\. Each point represents the odds ratio, and the lines extending left and right from each point represent the lower and upper confidence intervals, respectively.

Table 5. Results of a logistic regression model of dichotomized blood lead level (above or below 2µg/dL).

Pseudo R^2 = 0.1687

Variables	OR	p-value
Water Access at Birth	0.73	<0.0001
Year Tested	0.78	<0.0001
Black Population Fraction	1.81	<0.0001
Home Value (Log)	0.63	<0.0001
Gender	1.07	0.0063
Municipal Status	1.07	0.21
Hispanic Population Fraction	1.47	0.047
Median Household Income	1.00	0.30
Age		
18 to 36 Months	1.3	<0.0001
36 to 54 Months	1.1	0.03
Over 54 Months	1.3	0.43
Year Household Built		
1950 to 1970	0.64	<0.0001
1970 to 1990	0.54	<0.0001
1990 to 2000	0.44	<0.0001
2000 to 2005	0.39	<0.0001
After 2005	0.48	<0.0001
N	34314	

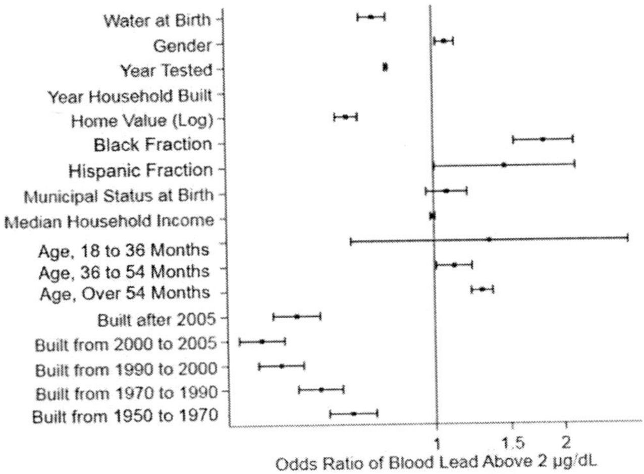

Figure 3. Graphical representation of the 2 µg/dL logistic model with odds ratios, confidence intervals, and all variables included in model. Each point represents the odds ratio, and the lines extending left and right from each point represent the lower and upper confidence intervals, respectively.

DISCUSSION

The objective of this study was to characterize the effects of exclusion from municipal water infrastructure on childhood blood lead levels in the community studied. We found that municipal water access and childhood blood lead levels are significantly associated across all models in this dataset. Children without municipal water access were more likely to have elevated blood lead levels as compared to children with municipal water access in the area studied. These findings support our hypothesis that a lack of access to municipal water is associated with elevated blood lead levels in our study population.

The findings of this study lend support to the hypothesis that private well water in underserved communities may contribute to the risk of elevated blood lead. Studies have found significant amounts of lead from private well water in neighborhoods without municipal water access in North Carolina (5). To date, this is the first study seeking to determine the relationship between a lack of municipal water access and childhood blood lead levels

Multiple studies have described racial disparities in municipal water access in North Carolina (8, 11, 13, 17, 18) and Wake County specifically (10). Predominantly Black communities in this area are significantly less likely to have municipal water access (10). Our results further these studies' findings by providing evidence that Black communities are also more likely to have elevated blood lead levels.

It is also important to consider the historical context of race in drawing municipal boundaries and providing municipal services in some communities. Predominantly Black communities have been historically excluded from municipal boundaries in some jurisdictions (6, 8, 13, 18). The results of this study suggest potential health risks associated with being excluded from municipal boundaries by increased blood lead levels due to unregulated private wells, especially for predominantly Black communities. Health effects from lead exposure in childhood include decreased IQ, poor school performance, and increased risk of delinquent behavior (2). The severe and pointed effects of childhood lead exposure are still an issue today, and drinking water constitutes a major source of lead exposure in some communities.

The findings of this study have many implications for public health and urban planning policy. Our results demonstrate a clear relationship between childhood blood lead levels and municipal water access. The results of this study demonstrate a clear relationship between demographics at the census block level and childhood blood lead levels. This demonstrated relationship in Wake County, while not generalizable to other locations, could be used by municipalities to determine which neighborhoods are most likely to benefit greatly from municipal water extensions.

Cycle of childhood environmental health disparities

Lead exposure in childhood is one example of persistent environmental health disparities experienced more frequently by communities of color. Figure 4 shows the cycle of childhood environmental health disparities experienced by communities without access to municipal water infrastructure. Children living in underbounded communities without access to public drinking water infrastructure rely on private wells, which are unregulated under the Safe Drinking Water Act. Public water systems governed by the Safe Drinking Water Act are required to implement corrosion controls to prevent the leaching of lead into the water supply, but private wells do not have these protections (15). Corrosive ground water from private wells can cause lead to leach from well and plumbing components (19).

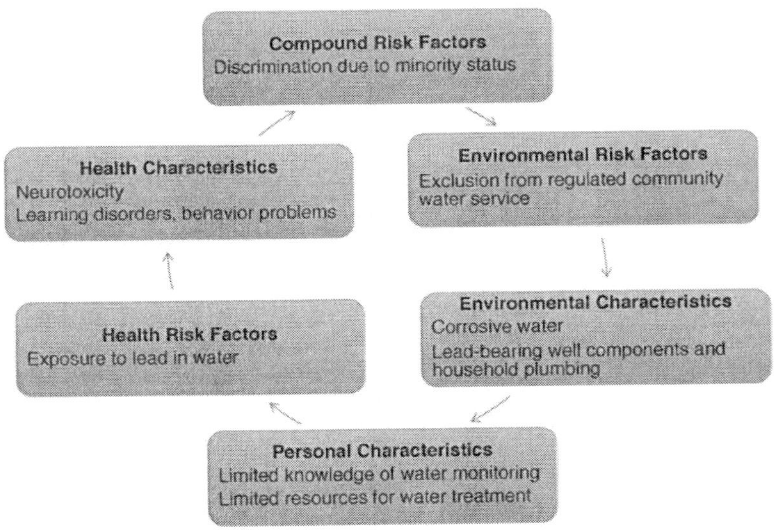

Figure 4. The cycle of childhood environmental health disparities experienced by individuals excluded from municipal water services due to racial underbounding of their community.

Households that rely on private wells are likely to neither have the knowledge nor the means to monitor water quality and/or to maintain their water systems should an issue be discovered (20–23). Thus, children living in these communities without access to municipal water infrastructure are at a greater risk for elevated blood lead levels, as demonstrated in this study's results. A report published by the CDC found blood lead levels of Black and Hispanic children were elevated compared to the blood lead levels of white children (1). Lead exposure in childhood results in negative health outcomes such as neurotoxicity, learning disorders, and behavioral problems, even at low levels of exposure (24–26). To break this cycle of childhood environmental health disparities, targeted interventions must be implemented to better educate private well owners on the importance of testing water quality regularly and implementing corrosion controls. Additionally, policy makers should work with historically underbounded communities to facilitate the extension of municipal water infrastructure.

Acknowledgments

We would like to thank the US EPA Science to Achieve Results program (grant number 83927901) for funding this research. We would also like to thank Jason Rotter and Philip McDaniel of the UNC Chapel Hill Odum Institute for assisting in the analysis of our data.

References

[1] Wheeler W, Brown MJ. Blood lead levels in children aged 1-5 years--United States, 1999-2010. MMWR 2013;62:245-8.

[2] Agency for Toxic Substances and Disease Registry. Toxicological profile for lead. Atlanta, GA: Agency for Toxic Substances and Disease Registry, 2019.

[3] Mushak P. Gastro-intestinal absorption of lead in children and adults: Overview of biological and biophysico-chemical aspects. Chem Speciat Bioavail 1991;3:87–104.

[4] Pieper KJ, Krometis LAH, Gallagher DL, Benham BL, Edwards M. Incidence of waterborne lead in private drinking water systems in Virginia. J Water Health 2015;13:897–908.

[5] Stillo FJ, MacDonald Gibson J. Racial disparities in access to municipal water supplies in the American South: impacts on children's health. Int Public Health J 2018;10(3):309-23.

[6] Aiken CCS. Race as a factor in municipal underbounding. Ann Assoc Am Geogr 1987;77:37–41.

[7] Lichter DT, Parisi D, Grice SM, Taquino M. Municipal underbounding: annexation and racial exclusion in small southern towns. Rural Sociol 2007;72:47–68.

[8] Parnell AM, Joyner AM, Christman CJ, Marsh DP. The persistence of political segregation: racial underbounding in North Carolina. Mebane, NC: Cedar Grove Institute Sustainable Communities, 2004.

[9] Durst NJ. Municipal annexation and the selective underbounding of colonias in Texas' Lower Rio Grande Valley. Environ Plan 2014;46:1699–1715.

[10] MacDonald Gibson J, DeFelice N, Sebastian D, Leker H. Racial disparities in access to community water supply service in Wake County, North Carolina. Am J Public Health 2014;104(12):e45.

[11] Leker HG, MacDonald Gibson J. Relationship between race and community water and sewer service in North Carolina, USA. PLoS One 2018;13:1–19.

[12] Wilson B, Edwards MM. Annexation and ethnicity in the American Midwest. Urban Aff Rev 2014;50:417–47.

[13] Johnson JH, Parnell A, Joyner AM, Christman CJ, Marsh B. Racial apartheid in a small North Carolina town. Rev. Black Polit. Econ 2004;31:89–107.

[14] Marsh B, Parnell AM, Joyner AM. Institutionalization of racial inequality in local political geographies. Urban Geogr 2010:31;691–709.

[15] US Congress. Safe drinking water act, 1974.

[16] American Academy of Pediatrics Committee on Environmental Health and Committee on Infectious Diseases. Drinking water from private wells and risks to children. Pediatrics 2009;123:1599–1605.

[17] Heaney CD, Wing S, Wilson SM, Campbell RL, Caldwell D, Hopkins B, et al. Public infrastructure disparities and the microbiological and chemical safety of drinking and surface water supplies in a community bordering a landfill. J Environ Health 2013;75:24–36.

[18] Joyner AM, Christman CJ. Segregation in the modern South? A case study of southern Moore County. Mebane, NC: Cedar Grove Institute Sustainable Communities, 2005.

[19] Pieper KJ, Krometis LA, Gallagher D, Benham B, Edwards M. Profiling private water systems to identify patterns of waterborne lead exposure. Environ Sci Technol 2015;49:12697-704.

[20] Roche SM, Jones-Bitton A, Majowicz SE, Pintar KDM, Allison D. Investigating public perceptions and knowledge translation priorities to improve water safety for residents with private water supplies: a cross-sectional study in Newfoundland and Labrador. BMC Public Health 2013;13:1225.

[21] Kreutzwiser R, de Loë R, Imgrund K, Conboy MJ, Simpson H, Plummer R. Understanding stewardship behaviour: factors facilitating and constraining private water well stewardship. J Environ Manage 2011;92:1104–14.

[22] Stillo FJ, Bruine de Bruin W, Zimmer C, MacDonald Gibson J. Well water testing in African American communities without municipal infrastructure: beliefs driving decisions. Environ Sci Technol 2019;686:1220-8.

[23] Fizer C, Bruine de Bruin W, Stillo FJ, MacDonald Gibson J. Barriers to managing private wells and septic systems in underserved communities: mental models of homeowner decision making. J. Environ. Health, In press.

[24] Lanphear BP, Hornung R, Ho M, Howard CR, Eberly S, Knauf K. Environmental lead exposure during early childhood. J Pediatr 2002;140:40–7.

[25] Lanphear BP, Hornung R, Khoury J, Yolton K, Baghurst P, Bellinger DC, et al. Low-level environmental lead exposure and children's intellectual function: an international pooled analysis. Environ Health Perspect 2005113:894–9.

[26] Searle AK, Baghurst PA, van Hooff M, Sawyer MG, Sim MR, Galletly C, et al. Tracing the long-term legacy of childhood lead exposure: a review of three decades of the Port Pirie Cohort study. Neurotoxicology 2014;43:46-56.

In: Child Environmental Health Disparities ISBN: 978-1-53617-823-4
Editors: IL Rubin and J Merrick © 2020 Nova Science Publishers, Inc.

Chapter 13

The Impact of Childhood Exercise and Household Income on Resilience in College Students

Leah Postilnik[1], BSN
and Maeve Howett[2,*], PhD, APRN, CPNP, IBCLC, CNE
[1] University of Massachusetts Amherst College of Nursing, Amherst, Massachusetts, United States of America
[2] Professor and Associate Dean for Baccalaureate Education, University of Maryland School of Nursing, Baltimore, Maryland, United States of America

Abstract

Living in poverty has detrimental effects on children's health. Children who are resilient may be protected from the damaging health effects of a low-income environment. There is a moderate amount of literature

* Correspondence: Maeve Howett, PhD, APRN, CPNP, IBCLC, CNE Professor and Associate Dean for Baccalaureate Education, University of Maryland School of Nursing, Office 404-H, 655 W. Lombard Street, Baltimore, MD 21201, 410-706-2156 United States. Email: mhowett@umaryland.edu.

suggesting exercise behaviors can increase resilience. In this study, we investigate whether college students from low-income environments with established childhood exercise habits are more resilient than students who exercised less. An electronic survey sent to students at the University of Massachusetts, Amherst included the Brief Resilience Scale© to measure students' resilience levels and the Godin Leisure-Time Exercise Questionnaire© to measure current and past exercise habits. The final analysis included 269 responses. Across income brackets, participants exercise most frequently in high school and least frequently in college. Students in the lowest household income bracket exercise the least while students from the highest household income bracket exercise the most. Students in the high-medium income bracket had the lowest mean resilience scores, and students in the highest income bracket had the highest resilience scores. When controlling for other variables, college exercise was shown to predict increased resilience scores. Additionally, middle school exercise was shown to predict high school and college exercise. These results demonstrate the necessity of interventions to increase exercise in children from low-income environments, establish exercise habits early in childhood, and use exercise as a strategy to promote resilience. Such interventions may enable children to protect themselves from developing chronic diseases caused by their environmental circumstances and thus break the cycle of environmental health disparities.

INTRODUCTION

Living in poverty has detrimental effects on children's health – children from low-income households have an increased risk of developing behavioral disorders (1) and developing a chronic disease later in life compared to children from higher income families (2). The list of possible underlying causes of these conditions is extensive – studies identify pollution (3), food insecurity (4), poor housing quality (5), lack of access to recreational space (6) and healthcare providers (7). These factors highlight the environmental health disparity between children from low-income households compared to average or high-income households. In order to mitigate the potential damaging health effects of poverty and break the cycle of health disparities, children need to have tools to manage increased stressors of their environment and cope with the adverse effects.

Frequent exercise has been shown to be one method that allows children to manage stress and improve their mental health (8). Since children in low-income environments experience higher stress levels (9) they may greatly benefit from using exercise to overcome the challenges of their harsh surroundings. Unfortunately, children from low-income households exercise significantly less than their wealthier peers (10). Research has identified a lack of access to recreational spaces (11), inadequate sports facilities (12) and unsafe neighborhood conditions (13) as possible causes of this disparity. The impact of children's physical environment on physical and mental health has become a highly researched subject, and the relationship may be more complicated than previously thought. For example, Huynh et al. (14) showed that children who reside near highways have a two-fold increased risk of uncontrolled asthma compared to children living more than two miles from a highway.

Developing resilience to the harsh environmental conditions associated with living in a low-income household would allow children to protect themselves the long-term damaging effects of asthma and other environmentally triggered conditions. The American Psychological Association (15) defines resilience as "the process of adapting well in the face of adversity, trauma, tragedy, threats or significant sources of stress." In a 2014 review of literature on the subject of resilience, Southwhick et al. (16) describe psychological resilience as complex construct with determinants that include "a host of biological, psychological, social and cultural factors that interact with one another to determine how one responds to stressful experiences." Studies have shown these factors to include emotional intelligence (17), self-esteem, number of adverse life experiences, and quality of parental relationships (18).

In this study, we measure the resilience of college students from different backgrounds and examine the role of past and present exercise habits as a factor in their resilience level. Based on literature that demonstrates the role of exercise in reducing stress and the protective nature of resilience (19,20), we hypothesize that established exercise habits will increase the resilience levels of children from low-income environments and bring them closer to breaking the cycle of health disparities (see Figure 1)

We decided to measure exercise habits over time in addition to current exercise patterns because we felt measuring long-term habits would yield an understanding of when interventions focused on exercise would be most effective in increasing resilience. Additionally, none of the previous literature on this subject explores the impact of long-term exercise habits and family income on resilience in college students specifically. Thus, our study will address this gap in the literature and yield a better understanding of how long-standing exercise habits impact college students' resilience levels and how family income impacts this relationship.

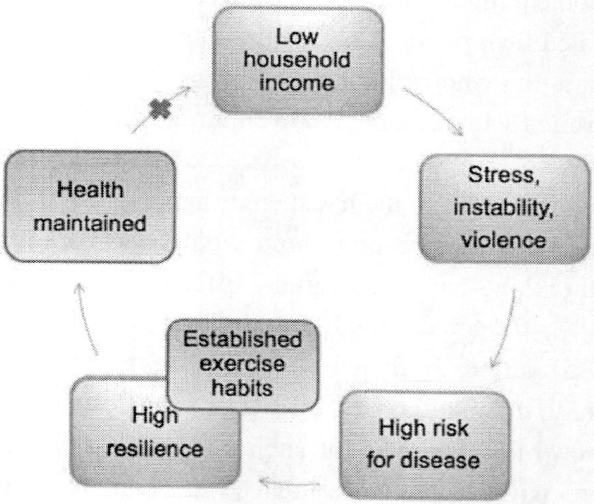

Figure 1. Hypothesis of the role of established exercise habits in breaking the cycle of health disparities.

OUR STUDY

This study was conducted at the University of Massachusetts (UMass), Amherst, a large four-year public institution. UMass Amherst is an appropriate setting for conducting this research due to the diverse student population; approximately one out of five students in the 2018 entering class are first generation college students and 15% of students are from underrepresented minority groups (21). After approval by the University's Institutional Review Board, a 23-question, five-minute, online electronic survey was developed using RedCap©, a HIPPA-compliant survey software. To recruit participants, the survey link was sent to 13 professors to forward to their class lists, posted on two class Facebook© pages, and verbally presented to students in three lectures halls at the beginning of that day's lecture.

Questionnaire

A single electronic survey was developed by combining the Brief Resilience Scale©, three iterations of the Godin-Shephard Leisure-Time Exercise Questionnaire© and participant demographic questions. Results from the Brief Resilience Scale allow researchers to assess respondents' resilience as "ability to bounce back from stress" and assign a unitary construct to resilience with as few queries as possible (22). This scale was chosen because it is a concise yet reliable method of quantifying resilience (22). The Godin-Shephard Leisure-Time Exercise Questionnaire© is a self-reported survey of weekly instances of mild, moderate, and strenuous leisure time exercise (23). In order to examine how exercise habits change over time, researchers included the survey three times, asking students about their exercise frequency in middle school, high school, and college. In addition to its high reliability and validity (24), the Godin-Shephard Leisure-Time Exercise Questionnaire© was chosen because it can be used to calculate a weighted exercise score based on the type of exercise. Researchers agree with the creator of the scale who states that the ability to weigh exercise by type provides a more comprehensive description of participants' exercise habits than scales that do not account for the type of exercise (23). Additionally, both questionnaires produce numerical results which were used for quantitative analysis.

Demographics

Demographic questions included age, gender, academic grade level, family household income, financial aid status, parental education level, and ability to cover household expenses. Yearly family household income was broken into four brackets: high ($200,000 or more), high-medium ($150,000-$199,999), low-medium ($60,000-$149,999), and low (less than $60,000). These brackets were created to straddle the average family household income of a UMass Amherst student, which is $120,000 (25). Each of these income brackets is significantly above the national poverty level; researchers chose the income brackets so the sample would be evenly distributed in order to make reliable conclusions about exercise and resilience for each group of respondents.

Resilience

Resilience was measured using the Brief Resilience Scale© developed by Smith et al. (22) in 2008 (Cronbach's alpha from .80 - .91 over four samples). This scale was chosen over the more extensive resilience scales in order to promote completion of the entire survey and increase the number of valid responses. The scale includes three positively worded statements such as "I tend to bounce back quickly after hard times" and three negatively worded statements such as "I have a hard time making it through stressful events" (22). Students respond to these statements on a Likert scale from Strongly Disagree to Strongly Agree. Based on responses to these statements, a resilience score was assigned to each participant on a scale from one to five.

Exercise habits

Long-term exercise habits were measured using a modified version of the Godin-Shephard Leisure-Time Exercise Questionnaire© (23). Independent evaluations of the scale have shown it to have satisfactory validity and reliability checks against gold-standard measures of physical activity (24). The original scale asks how many times per week participants perform mild, moderate and strenuous exercise at one point in time. The scale was modified and repeated three times, asking students about their exercise habits in middle school, high school, and college. To calculate a weighted exercise score for each time period, moderate exercise weekly instances were multiplied by two, and strenuous exercise weekly instances were multiplied by three and added to the other types of exercise. Additionally, a total exercise score was calculated by adding the weighted sums from the three time periods.

Data analysis

After the data collection period, quantitative statistical analysis with multiple regression was performed on SPSS software version 25© (26). A total of 300 surveys were submitted by participants. 31 surveys were not included in the analysis because respondents did not fill out the survey to completion. Resilience and exercise scores were averaged for participants in each of the four income brackets to examine correlations with income. For multiple regression analysis, a *p*-value of 0.05 was used to determine the statistical significance of relationships between demographic variables, resilience score, and exercise at each time period.

FINDINGS

Of the 269 surveys included in the final analysis, 73.2% percent of participants were female and 26.8% percent were male (see Table 1). Most participants (70.6%) reported receiving some form of financial aid. The largest group of participants (38.8%) were college juniors. Additionally, the largest group of respondents (42.8%) was in the low-medium income bracket. Most participants (71.4%) reported that one parent had at least a bachelor's degree (see Table 1 for demographic information).

Table 1. Participant demographics

Variable Label	*N*	Percent
Gender		
Female	197	73.2
Male	72	26.8
Age		
19	45	16.7
20	95	35.3
21	76	28.3
Older than 21	53	19.7
Year		
Freshman	16	5.9
Softmore	76	28.3
Junior	103	38.3
Senior	69	25.7
Other	5	1.9
Race		
American Indian or Native American	3	1.1
Asian or Pacific Islander	29	10.8
Black or African American	9	3.3
Caucasian (Non-Hispanic)	225	83.6
Hispanic	11	4.1
Other	9	3.3
Household Income		
Less than $60,000	31	11.5
$60,000 to $149999	115	42.8
$150,000 to $199,999	66	24.5
$200,000 or more	57	21.2
Ability to Cover Expenses		
Yes	232	86.2
No	14	5.2
Sometimes	23	8.6
Financial Aid Recipient		
Yes	190	70.6
No	79	29.4
Highest Parent Education		
Less than a high school diploma	1	0.4
High school degree or equivalent	22	8.2
Some college	27	10
Bachelor's degree	98	36.4
Master's degree or Doctorate degree	121	45

The distribution of mean exercise scores in middle school, high school, and college by income bracket is displayed in the graph titled *Exercise by household income level in middle school, high school and college* (see Figure 2).

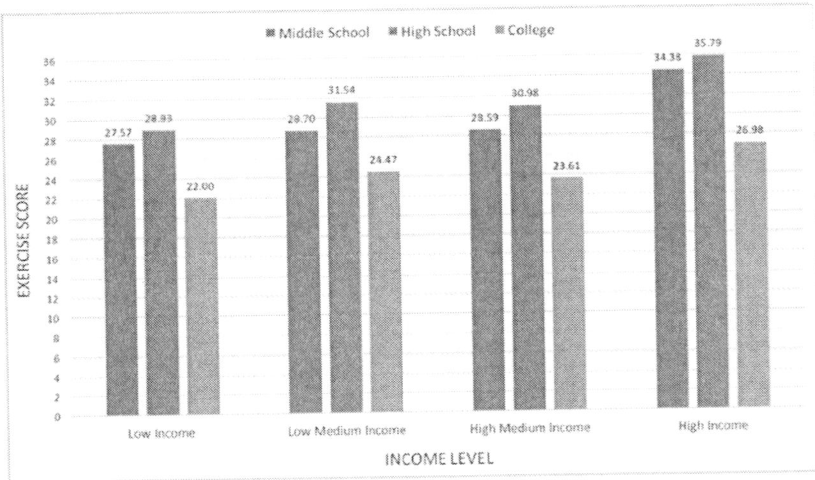

Figure 2. Exercise by household income level in middle school, high school and college.

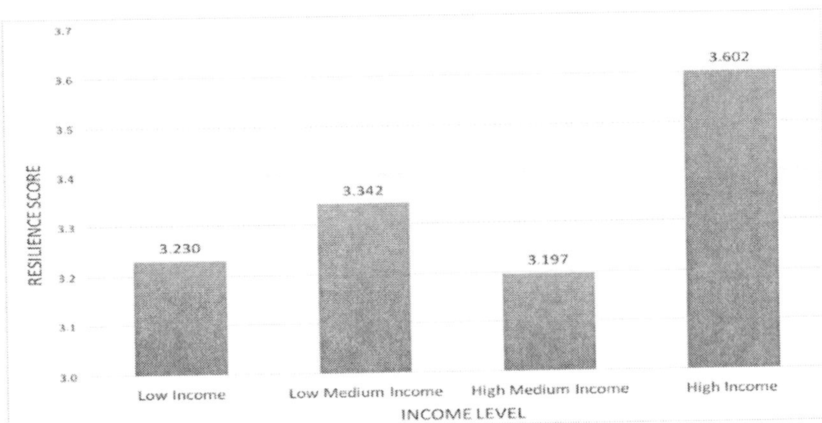

Figure 3. Mean resilience score by income level.

Across all income brackets, participants exercise most frequently in high school and least frequently in college. Exercise frequency was positively correlated with income level in all three time periods. Students in the lowest income bracket exercise the least in middle school, high school, and college, while students from the highest income bracket exercise the most. In addition to exercise, resilience was also lower among students in the lowest income bracket than the resilience of students in the highest bracket, but overall the relationship between income and resilience was not linear. Students in the high-medium income bracket had the lowest resilience scores. Mean resilience scores by income are displayed in the graph titled *Mean Resilience Score by Income level* (see Figure 3). The graph titled *Sum of individual exercise scores compared to individual mean resilience scores* shows participants' total exercise score (the sum of their weighted scores in middle school, high school, and college) compared to their resilience score (see Figure 4). While there is a large amount of variability in the results, there is a slight positive relationship between exercise and resilience. Multiple linear regression analysis showed that, when controlling for all other variables, exercise in college correlated with students' resilience score. Additionally, middle school exercise was shown to strongly predict high school exercise and moderately predict college exercise.

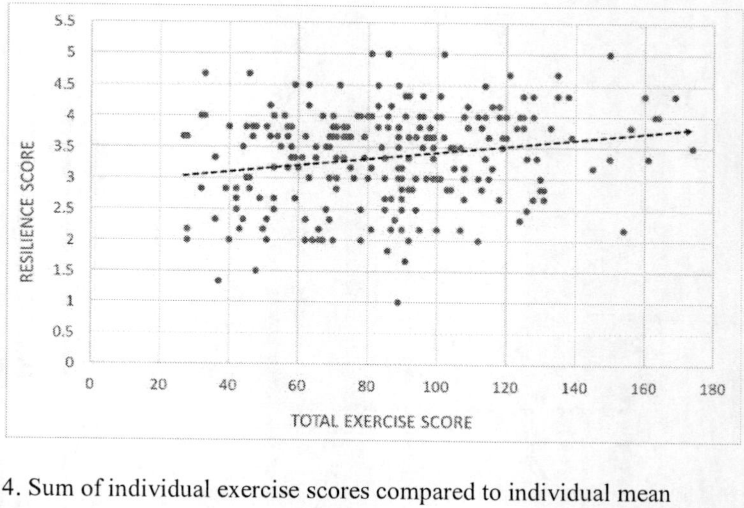

Figure 4. Sum of individual exercise scores compared to individual mean resilience scores.

Discussion

The purpose of this study was to measure whether childhood exercise habits impact the resilience of college students from different income levels. Respondents were divided into four income brackets. Students' resilience scores and weekly frequency of mild, moderate, and vigorous exercise levels in middle school, high school and college were analyzed. Trends and positive correlations in student's resilience and exercise seen in this study are consistent with current literature and can be used to make recommendations to increase resilience through exercise. The primary finding that college exercise was predictor of resilience in this dataset adds weight to the existing literature demonstrating a connection between exercise and resilience. The significance of this finding is increased by the fact that the largest percentage of participants were college juniors, who, by the third year of college, may have more consistent habits than freshmen. Although some students may have left the university by Junior year, 86.6% of UMass Amherst Juniors were retained from the original freshman class (27). The relationship between frequent exercise and increased resilience can be used to support the implementation of exercise programs targeted towards increasing resilience and improving mental health of college students. The finding that students who exercise in middle school continue to exercise in high school and college reveals exercise habits are established early in life and is consistent with literature on the subject. Thus, we recommend interventions for children across income levels should begin with introducing exercise at a young age since the habit will likely be maintained in young adulthood and beyond.

While individual interventions are important, local and national governments should also recognize the impact of environmental improvements on exercise outcomes of entire communities. A greenway built in Knoxville, Tennessee significantly increased the amount of time community members spent walking and biking (28), although other studies show that trail users are most likely to be white adult males (29). Among children from low-income households in Chicago, perceived neighborhood safety was associated with the amount of unstructured play while access to neighborhood exercise facilities predicted organized sport participation (30). Healthcare policy advocates should refer to case studies and literature that demonstrates the impact of green space, recreational facilities and safe neighborhoods on children's health to promote policies that improve the built environment.

When controlling for other variables with multiple regression analysis, family income and other socioeconomic variables did not significantly predict resilience or exercise. Although student demographics did not predict exercise habits in the data, there was a positive correlation between exercise and income level. This finding is consistent with the robust literature demonstrating the disparity in exercise habits of children in low and high-income environments (31). Trends in resilience by income were less linear – students in the high-medium income bracket had lower resilience scores than students in the two lower income brackets. Studies of childhood development and stress have shown that experiences of severe adversity, called ACEs (Adverse Childhood Experiences), have long-term destructive effects on children's physical and mental health (32). However, experiencing a moderate amount of adversity (as the students in the lower income levels most likely have) can contribute to the development of resilience (33). In a longitudinal survey of 1,994 participants, Seery et al. (33) found that respondents with a history of some lifetime adversity were less affected by adverse experiences than individuals with an extensive history of adversity or no history of adversity. Seery et al. (33) hypothesized that experiencing some adversity could "teach effective coping skills, help engage social support networks, create a sense of mastery over past adversity, foster beliefs in the ability to cope successfully in the future, and generate psychophysiological toughness" (33). The beneficial effect of moderate adversity can be compared to the common belief that strenuous exercise and sports "build character" (34). The literature on exercise and adversity suggests exercise may be a form of intentionally induced moderate adversity that creates a similar effect to the moderate stress described by Seery et al. (33). Further research should be conducted to compare the impact of experiencing purposeful, positive adversity through exercise to the impact of experiencing unfortunate adversity such as ACE's. Exercise may provide an opportunity for children to safely experience hardship and failure to develop psychological resilience that becomes vital when more serious challenges arise.

At the Mindfulness-Based Stress Reduction Clinic, located a short drive away from the UMass Amherst campus, students can learn resilience not only on the sports field, but also in a classroom. Participants practice mindfulness techniques which demonstrate that "paying attention on purpose, in the present moment, and nonjudgmentally, to the unfolding of experience moment to moment" can even help to manage physical conditions such as asthma, fibromyalgia, skin disorders and heart disease (35). This approach stresses the relationship between physiological habits and mental health. This mind-body relationship suggests that both physical and psychological training through exercise, meditation, and mindfulness, are important elements in fostering resilience for individuals of all ages.

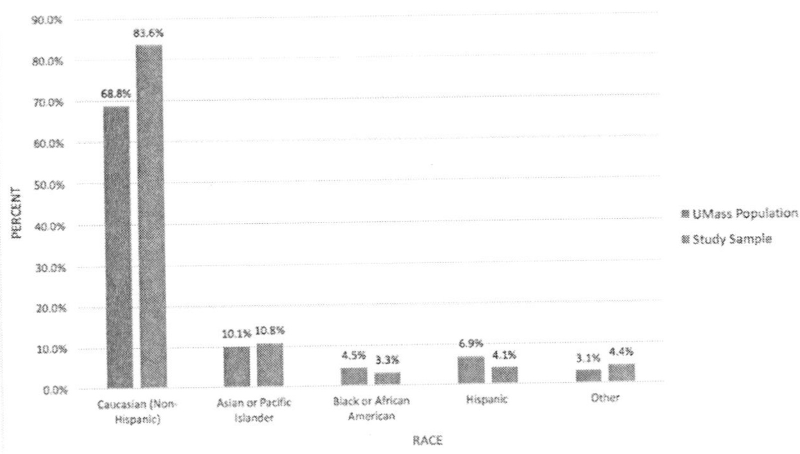

Figure 5. Race distribution of UMass student population versus study sample.

Limitations

Limitations of this study include the fact that the sample (n = 269) was relatively small, and from only one public university. The ethnic distribution of participants was representative of the UMass student population (see Figure 5), but due to the sample size the number of participants from minority groups was too small to be able to make conclusions about exercise and resilience of different ethnic groups. Additionally, students were mostly recruited from traditional lectures in disciplines such as computer science, business administration, nursing, biology, and engineering. Including students studying art, dance, or agricultural studies may be underrepresented because they do not attend traditional lectures and were therefore harder to recruit for this study. The unequal gender distribution of the sample (73.2% female) is likely due to the fact that one of the lectures researchers attended to recruit participants was a Nursing lecture and included mostly female students. In order to encourage completion of the entire survey, demographic questions were kept as concise and simple as possible, which may have resulted in loss of detail about students' backgrounds. Because participation was optional, the study population was self selecting, so results do not necessarily reflect information about other college students. The relatively high household income of the study population limits the study's generalizability. Future surveys should include an analysis of a more diverse sample as well as other socioeconomic variables in addition to income. A deeper exploration of students' lifestyle would be valuable – one suggestion is to ask students if they have to work to finance their education or pay back large student loans. Additionally, a longitudinal study that follows a cohort over time would be more accurate than retrospective responses. Finally, different methods of quantifying exercise habits, including real-time activity monitors such as watches or chest straps, would be useful to remove the inaccuracies of the self-reports used in this study.

CONCLUSION

Through a self-selected survey of college students, psychological resilience levels, family household income, and past and present exercise habits, student's exercise frequency was determined to predict students' resilience and that students who start exercising in middle school are likely to continue exercising in high school and in college. Results also showed household income level is directly related to how much a student exercises. The finding of a correlation between the low resilience and the poor exercise habits of children from low-income households shown in this study suggests exercise interventions should be targeted towards children in low-income environments to help them build resilience to the health risk factors that are prevalent in these environments. Furthermore, the relationship between exercise and resilience shown in this study should prompt health policy changes to improve children's environments making exercise accessible and safe in the critical middle school years, thereby promoting protective resilience against environmental stressors. Resilience built through holistic interventions that include consistent physical and psychological training will enable children to disrupt the cycle of health disparities resulting in improved health, educational achievement and success in life.

References

[1] Rubin IL, Geller RJ, Martinuzzi K, Howett M, Gitterman BA, Wells L, et al. Children's environmental health disparities: The costs and benefits of breaking the cycle. Int J Child Health Hum Dev 2016;9(4):419-30.

[2] Johnson RC, Schoeni RF. Early-life origins of adult disease: National longitudinal population-based study of the United States. Am J Public Health 2011;101(12):2317-24.

[3] Brulle RJ, Pellow DN. Environmental justice: Human health and environmental inequalities Annu Rev Public Health 2006;27:103–24.

[4] Bhattacharya J, Currie J, Haider S. Poverty, food insecurity, and nutritional outcomes in children and adults. J Health Econ 2004;23(4):839–62.

[5] Adamkiewicz G, Spengler JD, Harley, AE, Stoddard A, Yang M, Alvarez-Reeves M et al. Environmental conditions in low-income urban housing: Clustering and associations with self-reported health. Am J Public Health 2014;104(9):1650–56.

[6] Dahmann N, Wolch J, Joassart-Marcelli P, Reynolds K, Jerrett M. The active city? Disparities in provision of urban public recreation resources. Health Place 2010;16(3):431–45.

[7] Xingyou Z, Phillips Jr RL, Bazemore AW, Dodoo MS, Petterson SM, Xierall I et al Physician distribution and access: Workforce priorities. Am Fam Physician 2008;77(10):1378.

[8] Geertsen SS, Thomas R, Larsen MN, Dahn IM, Andersen JN, Krause-Jensen M, et al. Motor skills and exercise capacity are associated with objective measures of cognitive functions and academic performance in preadolescent children. PLoS One 2016;11(8):e0161960. doi: 10.1371/journal.pone.0161960.

[9] Finegood ED, Wyman C, O'Connor TG, Blair CB. Salivary cortisol and cognitive development in infants from low-income communities. Stress 2017;20:112–21.

[10] Jin Y, Jones-Smith JC. Associations between family income and children's physical fitness and obesity in California, 2010-2012. Prev Chronic Dis 2015;12 :140392. doi: http://dx.doi.org/10.5888/pcd12.140392.

[11] Schalkwijk AA, Zwaard BC, Nijpels G, Elders PJ, Platt L. The impact of greenspace and condition of the neighbourhood on child overweight. Eur J Public Health 2017;2:88-94.

[12] Black N, Johnston DW, Propper C, Shields MA. The effect of school sports facilities on physical activity, health and socioeconomic status in adulthood. Soc Sci Med 2019;220:120-8.

[13] Dias A, Gaya A, Brand C, Pizarro A, Fochesatto C, Mendes T, et al. Distance from home to the nearest park and the use of the parks for physical activity: The mediator role of road safety perception in adolescents. Am J Public Health 2019;168:9-16.

[14] Huynh P, Salam MT, Morphew T, Kwong KY, Scott L. Residential proximity to freeways is associated with uncontrolled asthma in inner-city Hispanic children and adolescents. J Allergy (Cairo) 2010;2010. Pii:157249. doi: 10.1155/2010/157249.

[15] American Psychological Association. The road to resilience. Washington, DC: APA, 2018. URL: http://www.apa.org/helpcenter/road-resilience.aspx.

[16] Southwick SM, Bonanno, GA, Masten AS, Panter-Brick, C, Yehuda R. Resilience definitions, theory, and challenges: Interdisciplinary perspectives. Eur J Psychotraumatol 2014;5:10.3402/ejpt.v5.25338. doi: 10.3402/ejpt.v5.25338.

[17] Armstrong R, Galligan RF, Critchley CR. Emotional intelligence and psychological resilience to negative life events. Pers Individ Diff 2011;51(3):331-6.

[18] Edwards T, Catling JC, Perry E. Identifying predictors of resilience in children. Psychol Teach Rev 2016;22(1):26-34.

[19] Lee SW, Bae GY, Rim HD, Lee SJ, Chang SM, Kim BS, et al. Mediating effect of resilience on the association between emotional neglect and depressive symptoms. Psychiatr Investig 2018;15(1):62-9.

[20] Shi J, Chen Z, Yin F, Zhao J, Zhao X, Yao, Y. Resilience as moderator of the relationship between left-behind experience and mental health of Chinese adolescents. Int J Soc Psychiatry 2016;62(4):386-93.

[21] Diversity Matters. University of Massachusetts Amherst 2019. URL: https://www.umass.edu/diversity/data-policies.

[22] Smith BW, Dalen J, Wiggins K, Tooley E, Christopher P, Bernard J. The brief resilience scale: Assessing the ability to bounce back. Int J Behav Med 2008;15(3):194-200.

[23] Godin G. The godin-shephard leisure-time physical activity questionnaire. CMAJ 2011;4(1):18-22.
[24] Hagger MS, Chatzisarantis NL, Barkoukis V, Wang CK, Baranowski J. Perceived autonomy support in physical education and leisure-time physical activity: A cross-cultural evaluation of the trans-contextual model. J Educ Psychol 2005;97(3):376-90.
[25] University of Massachusetts Amherst. National Center for Education Statistics 2019 URL: https://nces.ed.gov/collegenavigator/?id=166629#finaid.
[26] IBM Corp. IBM SPSS statistics for windows, version 25.0. Armonk, NY: IBM, 2017.
[27] University of Massachusetts Amherst. Retention and graduation rates of entering full-time first-year students fall 2008-fall 2017. University of Massachusetts Amherst Office of Institutional Research. URL: https://www.umass.edu/oir/sites/default/files/publications/factsheets/retention/FS_ret_03.pdf.
[28] Fitzhugh EC, Bassett Jr DR, Evans MF. Urban trails and physical activity: A natural experiment. Am J Prev Med 2010;39(3):259-62.
[29] Reed JA, Hooker SP, Muthukrishnan S, Hutto B. User demographics and physical activity behaviors on a newly constructed urban rail/trail conversion. J Phys Act Health 2011;8(4):534-42.
[30] Appelhans BM, Li H. organized sports and unstructured active play as physical activity sources in children from low-income, Chicago households. Pediatr Exerc Sci 2016; 28(3):381-7.
[31] Drenowatz C, Eisenmann JC, Pfeiffer KA, Welk G, Heelan K, Gentile D, Walsh D. Influence of socio-economic status on habitual physical activity and sedentary behavior in 8- to 11-year old children. BMC Public Health 2010;10:214.
[32] Hughes K, Bellis MA, Hardcastle KA, Sethi D, Butchart A, Mikton C, et al. The effect of multiple adverse childhood experiences on health: A systematic review and meta-analysis. Lancet Public Health 2017;2(8):e356-66.
[33] Seery MD, Holman EA, Silver RC. Whatever does not kill us: Cumulative lifetime adversity, vulnerability, and resilience. J Pers Soc Psychol 2010;99(6):1025-41.
[34] Gerber M, Kalak N, Lemola S, Clough PJ, Pühse U, Elliot C, Holsboer-Trachsler E, Brand S. Adolescents' exercise and physical activity are associated with mental toughness. Ment Health Phys Act 2012;(5)1:35-42.
[35] Center for Mindfulness. Journal Articles and Publications. URL: https://www.umassmed.edu/cfm/mindfulness-based-programs/mbsr-courses/about-mbsr/mbsr-journal-articles/.

SECTION THREE: ACKNOWLEDGMENTS

In: Child Environmental Health Disparities ISBN: 978-1-53617-823-4
Editors: IL Rubin and J Merrick

Chapter 14

About the Editors

I Leslie Rubin, MD, is originally from South Africa where he trained in pediatrics and emigrated to the United States in 1976. He is currently Associate Professor in the Department of Pediatrics at Morehouse School of Medicine, Adjunct Associate Professor, Department of Pediatrics, Emory University School of Medicine, Co-director of the Southeast Pediatric Environmental Health Unit at Emory University, President and Founder or Break the Cycle of Health Disparities Inc, and Medical Director of The Rubin Center for Autism and Developmental Pediatric in Atlanta, Georgia. He has been involved in the health care of children and adults with intellectual and developmental disabilities since 1977. In 1989, he and Allen Crocker published the first textbook on medical care for children and adults with developmental disabilities. Sadly, Allen Crocker passed away in 2011, but, in partnership with Joav Merrick and others published the 3rd edition: "Health care for people with intellectual and developmental disabilities across the lifespan" by Springer 2016. He currently directs interdisciplinary clinical programs for children with autism, cerebral palsy and other developmental disabilities and consults to a variety of programs including the Emory University Neurodevelopmental Exposure Clinic, which is an interdisciplinary, research based program looking at the impact of prenatal exposures on child development and behavior in the context of the social and economic disadvantage and health disparities. Among his awards for various activities, he received the Robert E. Cooke Lifetime Achievement Award from the AADMD in 2015 and the Autism Achievement Award in 2016 from the Annual Conference and Exposition of Georgia, and the F Edwards Rushton CATCH Award from the American Academy of Pediatric in 2018. He is actively involved in the American Academy of Pediatrics as the Chair of the Environmental Health Committee and District X CATCH Facilitator for the AAP. He is on the US Environmental Protection Agency Board of Scientific Counsellors focusing on Sustainable Healthy Communities. He is also the Chair of the National PEHSU Steering Committee and is on the Advisory Councils of HERCULES, the Human Exposome Reach Center; CCHEM, the Children's Environmental Health Research Center; and the Center of Excellence in Maternal and Child Health Education, Science, and Practice, all at Emory University and on the National START Advisory Committee based at the University of New Hampshire. In 2004, he started the Break the Cycle programs and founded Break the Cycle of Health Disparities, Inc to focus on Break the Cycle of Environmental Health Disparities now in its 15th year. The program received the Children's Environmental Health Excellence Award from the EPA in 2016. Email: lrubi01@emory.edu

Joav Merrick, MD, MMedSci, DMSc, born and educated in Denmark is professor of pediatrics, Division of Pediatrics, Hadassah Hebrew University Medical Center, Mt Scopus Campus, Jerusalem, Israel and Kentucky Children's Hospital, University of Kentucky, Lexington, Kentucky United States and professor of public health at the Center for Healthy Development, School of Public Health, Georgia State University, Atlanta, United States, the former medical director of the Health Services, Division for Intellectual and Developmental Disabilities, Ministry of Social Affairs and Social Services, Jerusalem, the founder and director of the National Institute of Child Health and Human Development in Israel. Numerous publications in the field of pediatrics, child health and human development, rehabilitation, intellectual disability, disability, health, welfare, abuse, advocacy, quality of life and prevention. Received the Peter Sabroe Child Award for outstanding work on behalf of Danish Children in 1985 and the International LEGO-Prize ("The Children's Nobel Prize") for an extraordinary contribution towards improvement in child welfare and well-being in 1987. In 2017 appointed a Kentucky Colonel by the Commonwealth of Kentucky, the highest honor the governor can bestow to a person. Email: jmerrick@zahav.net.il

In: Child Environmental Health Disparities ISBN: 978-1-53617-823-4
Editors: IL Rubin and J Merrick

Chapter 15

About the Break the Cycle of Health Disparities Inc

Break the Cycle of Health Disparities Inc is a private, not-for-profit 501c3 or non-governmental organization dedicated to exploring the social economic and environmental determinants of health in the context of children's health disparities and to use this to promote health equity for all children.

Break the Cycle of Health Disparities Inc collaborates with the Southeast PEHSU to produce the annual Break the Cycle of Children's Environmental Health Disparities Program (Break the Cycle). Break the Cycle is a multidisciplinary academic program that focuses on raising awareness of children's environmental health disparities and cultivating future leaders among university students in the fields of medicine, nursing, public health, law, social work, education and other related disciplines.

Each year, Break the Cycle invites students from a diversity of colleges and universities to develop projects that will "break the cycle of children's environmental health disparities". The students present their completed projects at a national conference and their work is published in international journals. Over the past 14 years Break the Cycle has engaged over 120 students from 30 different university departments in 10 states in the USA, as well as students from Latin America, Europe and Africa, that have resulted in the publication of 11 journal supplements. These sets of projects form the basis for this book series.

In 2016, Break the Cycle received a Children's Environmental Health Excellence Award from the US Environmental Protection Agency for the achievements of the program.

Contact

I Leslie Rubin MD
Associate Professor, Department of Pediatrics,
Morehouse School of Medicine
Adjuct Associate Profesor, Department of Pediatrics,
Emory University School of Medicine
Co-director, Southeast Pediatric Environmental Health Specialty Unit,
Emory University School of Medicine
President and Founder, Break the Cycle of Health Disparities Inc
Medical Director, The Rubin Center for Autism and
Developmental Pediatrics
750 Hammond Drive, Building 1, Suite 100, Atlanta, GA 30328,
United States
Email: lrubi01@emory.edu
Website: www.breakthecycleprogram.org
Website: www.pehsu.emory.edu
Website: www.therubincenterfor autism.org

In: Child Environmental Health Disparities ISBN: 978-1-53617-823-4
Editors: IL Rubin and J Merrick

Chapter 16

About the Pediatric Environmental Health Specialty Units (PEHSU)

The Pediatric Environmental Health Specialty Units (PEHSU's) are an interconnected system of regional centers located throughout the United States, that respond to questions from public health professionals, clinicians, policy makers, and the public about environmental health concerns related to children and reproductive age adults. After fifteen years of programmatic operations, collaborations, and and a growing desire to protect the health of children and reproductive age adults from environmental hazards, the PEHSU Program has gained the attention and respect of the pediatric and reproductive environmental medical community and families at risk from exposure to environmental contaminants. The PEHSU programs have a critical role in supporting the mission of the Agency for Toxic Substances and Disease Registry (ATSDR) to prevent or mitigate the adverse human health effects and diminished quality of life that result from exposure to hazardous substances in the environment, and the mission of the US Environmental Protection Agency (EPA) to protect human health and the environment. The PEHSUs provide a credible, academic, non-commercial source of health information and clinical expertise regarding environmental toxins and their effects on children and reproductive age adults.

ATSDR and EPA established the PEHSUs to increase the capacity of health care providers to identify and treat environmental-related health conditions, prevent exposure to children and reproductive age adults, and communicate health risks from environmental exposures. The PEHSU Network includes teams of medical specialists (pediatricians, medical toxicologists, epidemiologists, obstetricians, nurses, nurse practictioners, occupational and environmental health physicians), public health academics and professionals, psychologists and educators, in providing consultation, training, referrals and clinical services to health care providers, governmental agencies and the general public on pediatric and reproductive environmental health.

The National PEHSU Network helps individuals and communities with health-related decision-making on important areas of environmental health. The most common five exposures of concern, based on inquiries to the National PEHSU network from 2007 to 2011, were related to lead poisoning, fungus or mold, mercury, pesticides, phthalates and bisphenol A. There have also been responses generated around major public health concerns such as wildfires, hurricanes, oil spills, carbon monoxide, chelation, and other dramatic environmental crises like mercury spills, de-icer leaks at airports and industrial pollution in cities and towns. For example, PEHSUs have advised about optimal strategies in assessing the severity of exposure to chemicals of concern in air, water, and soil, as to whether blood or urine testing may be helpful and, if so, which tests are best obtained.

While Poison Control Centers respond to acute toxic exposures, the PEHSU Network has expertise in longer term, chronic lower dose exposures, group exposures, and the development and dissemination of appropriate public messages when needed. The PEHSU Network partners closely with local, state, and federal agencies and non-profit professional organizations in carrying out this work.

The PEHSUs have collaborated with ATSDR and EPA to develop fact sheets targeting clinicians and the public on issues associated with flooding, hurricanes, wildfires, oil spills, formaldehyde, carbon monoxide poisoning, arsenic in foods, medical management of lead exposure, phthalates and bisphenl A, melamine, and other issues. They have edited books, written articles, and conducted programming to give health professionals and the public a better understanding of pediatric envronmental medicine and environmental health on topics including:

- Indoor air contamination at home
- Hazards of living near toxic waste sites
- Inquiries about potential toxins, such as residential pesticides, childhood lead, well water contamination
- Daycare and preschool hazards
- School-related hazards
- Adolescent work place exposures
- Environmental health disparities and environmental justice

The PEHSU's also provide information via the internet (website www.pehsu.net) with a variety of materials, educating professionals in reproductive and children's environmental health through conferences presentations and formal university-based training programs and media outreach to inform the public about the facts of topics of relevance to environmental health. All PEHSU members serve on boards and committees to advance collaborative activities and community expertise in environmental health issues. The PEHSUs train and mentor medical, toxicology and other graduate students and residents from medical and public health schools, and provide training opportunities in pediatric environmental medicane and reproductive epidemiology. The PEHSUs have counselled first responders, parents, health officials, and school administrators on how to assess and rectify the damage from spills and other environmental emergencies. They have also provided training to establish PEHSUs in Chile, Argentina, Canada, Mexico, Vietnam, and Israel.

The PEHSUs d serve to translate research findings into clinical and public health practice. This program is an integral component in the development of healthcare professionals who are better prepared to recognize, treat, and prevent toxic environmental exposures in children.

Southeast PEHSU

The Southeast PEHSU, one of the network of US PEHSUs, serves the southeastern states of the United States: Alabama, North Carolina, South Carolina, Florida, Georgia, Kentucky, Mississippi and Tennessee. The Southeast PEHSU is based in the Department of Pediatrics at Emory University in Atlanta and works closely with Region 4 of the US Environmental Protection Agency (EPA) and the Agency for Toxic Substances and Disease Registry (ATSDR) at the Centers for Disease Control and Prevention (CDC). The team includes Robert J. Geller, MD (pediatric toxicologist), Leslie Rubin, MD (developmental pediatrician), Abby D. Mutic, BS, MSN, PhD (Certified Nurse Midwife), Victoria Green, MD, MHSA, JD, MBA (obstetrician), Claire Coles, PhD (psychologist), Nathan Mutic, MS (educator and program administrator), and Wayne Garfinkel, BSCE (formerly of Region 4 EPA). In adddition, Benjamin Gitterman, MD (pediatrician at Georgetown University in Washington DC) works with the Southeast PEHSU on the *Break the Cycle* programs. The Southeast PEHSU collaborates with the Break the Cycle of Health Disparities, Inc, to produce the *Break the Cycle* programs.

Contact Southeast PEHSU

Robert J Geller, MD
Director, Pediatric Environmental Health Specialty Unit
Emory University Department of Pediatrics
49 Jesse Hill Jr Drive SE, Atlanta, GA 30303, United States.
Toll free tel: (877) 33 PEHSU or (877) 337-3478
Tel: (404) 727-9428
Fax: (404) 616-6657
E-mail: rgeller@emory.edu
Website: www.pehsu.emory.edu

In: Child Environmental Health Disparities ISBN: 978-1-53617-823-4
Editors: IL Rubin and J Merrick

Chapter 17

About the National Institute of Child Health and Human Development in Israel

The National Institute of Child Health and Human Development (NICHD) in Israel was established in 1998 as a virtual institute under the auspices of the Medical Director, Ministry of Social Affairs and Social Services in order to function as the research arm for the Office of the Medical Director. In 1998 the National Council for Child Health and Pediatrics, Ministry of Health and in 1999 the Director General and Deputy Director General of the Ministry of Health endorsed the establishment of the NICHD.

Mission

The mission of a National Institute for Child Health and Human Development in Israel is to provide an academic focal point for the scholarly interdisciplinary study of child life, health, public health, welfare, disability, rehabilitation, intellectual disability and related aspects of human development. This mission includes research, teaching, clinical work information and public service activities in the field of child health and human development.

Service and academic activities

Over the years many activities became focused in the south of Israel due to collaboration with various professionals at the Faculty of Health Sciences (FOHS) at the Ben Gurion University of the Negev (BGU). Since 2000 an affiliation with the Zusman Child Development Center at the Pediatric Division of Soroka University Medical Center has resulted in collaboration around the establishment of the Down Syndrome Clinic at that center. In 2002 a full course on "Disability" was established at the Recanati School for Allied Professions in the Community, FOHS, BGU and in 2005 collaboration was started with the Primary Care Unit of the faculty and disability became part of the master of public health course on "Children and society". In the academic year 2005-2006 a one semester course on "Aging with disability" was started as part of the master of science program in gerontology in our collaboration with the Center for Multidisciplinary Research in Aging. In 2010 collaborations with the Division of Pediatrics, Hadassah Hebrew University Medical Center, Jerusalem, Israel around the National Down Syndrome Center and teaching students and residents about intellectual and developmental disabilities as part of their training at this campus.

Research activities

The affiliated staff have over the years published work from projects and research activities in this national and international collaboration. In the year 2000 the International Journal of Adolescent Medicine and Health and in 2005 the International Journal on Disability and Human Development of De Gruyter Publishing House (Berlin and New York) were affiliated with the National Institute of Child Health and Human Development. From 2008 also the International Journal of Child Health and Human Development (Nova Science, New York), the International Journal of Child and Adolescent Health (Nova Science) and the Journal of Pain Management (Nova Science) affiliated and from 2009 the International Public Health Journal (Nova

Science) and Journal of Alternative Medicine Research (Nova Science). All peer-reviewed international journals.

National collaborations

Nationally the NICHD works in collaboration with the Faculty of Health Sciences, Ben Gurion University of the Negev; Department of Physical Therapy, Sackler School of Medicine, Tel Aviv University; Autism Center, Assaf HaRofeh Medical Center; National Rett and PKU Centers at Chaim Sheba Medical Center, Tel HaShomer; Department of Physiotherapy, Haifa University; Department of Education, Bar Ilan University, Ramat Gan, Faculty of Social Sciences and Health Sciences; College of Judea and Samaria in Ariel and in 2011 affiliation with Center for Pediatric Chronic Diseases and National Center for Down Syndrome, Department of Pediatrics, Hadassah Hebrew University Medical Center, Mount Scopus Campus, Jerusalem.

International collaborations

Internationally with the Department of Disability and Human Development, College of Applied Health Sciences, University of Illinois at Chicago; Strong Center for Developmental Disabilities, Golisano Children's Hospital at Strong, University of Rochester School of Medicine and Dentistry, New York; Centre on Intellectual Disabilities, University of Albany, New York; Centre for Chronic Disease Prevention and Control, Health Canada, Ottawa; Chandler Medical Center and Children's Hospital, Kentucky Children's Hospital, Section of Adolescent Medicine, University of Kentucky, Lexington; Chronic Disease Prevention and Control Research Center, Baylor College of Medicine, Houston, Texas; Division of Neuroscience, Department of Psychiatry, Columbia University, New York; Institute for the Study of Disadvantage and Disability, Atlanta; Center for Autism and Related Disorders, Department Psychiatry, Children's Hospital Boston

Boston; Department of Pediatric and Adolescent Medicine, Western Michigan University Homer Stryker MD School of Medicine, Kalamazoo, Michigan, United States; Department of Paediatrics, Child Health and Adolescent Medicine, Children's Hospital at Westmead, Westmead, Australia; International Centre for the Study of Occupational and Mental Health, Düsseldorf, Germany; Centre for Advanced Studies in Nursing, Department of General Practice and Primary Care, University of Aberdeen, Aberdeen, United Kingdom; Quality of Life Research Center, Copenhagen, Denmark; Nordic School of Public Health, Gottenburg, Sweden, Scandinavian Institute of Quality of Working Life, Oslo, Norway; The Department of Applied Social Sciences (APSS) of The Hong Kong Polytechnic University Hong Kong.

Targets

Our focus is on research, international collaborations, clinical work, teaching and policy in health, disability and human development and to establish the NICHD as a permanent institute in Israel in order to conduct model research and provide policy aspects in the field of interest.

Contact

Professor Joav Merrick, MD, MMedSci, DMSc
Director, National Institute of Child Health and Human Development, Jerusalem, Israel. E-mail: jmerrick@zahav.net.il

SECTION FOUR: INDEX

INDEX

A

J

L

M